BUILDING AN AGELESS MIND

BUILDING AN AGELESS MIND

Preventing and Fighting Brain Aging and Disease

William J. Tippett

ROWMAN & LITTLEFIELD PUBLISHERS, INC.
Lanham • Boulder • New York • Toronto • Plymouth, UK

Published by Rowman & Littlefield Publishers, Inc.
A wholly owned subsidiary of The Rowman & Littlefield Publishing Group, Inc.
4501 Forbes Boulevard, Suite 200, Lanham, Maryland 20706
www.rowman.com

10 Thornbury Road, Plymouth PL6 7PP, United Kingdom

British Library Cataloguing in Publication Information Available

Library of Congress Cataloging-in-Publication Data

Tippett, William J., 1974– .
Building an ageless mind : preventing and fighting brain aging and disease / William J. Tippett.
p. cm.
Includes bibliographical references and index.
ISBN 978-1-4422-2048-5 (cloth : alk. paper) — ISBN 978-1-4422-2049-2 (electronic)
1. Brain—Diseases—Prevention—Popular works. 2. Brain—Aging—Prevention—Popular works. 3. Memory disorders—Prevention—Popular works. I. Title.
RC386.2.T57 2013
616.805—dc23
2013000227

Printed in the United States of America

To Jennifer, Abigail, Myles, and Declan. Thank you for unconditional love and support.

One should not pursue goals that are easily achieved. One must develop an instinct for what one can just barely achieve through one's greatest efforts. —Albert Einstein

CONTENTS

DISCLAIMER

This book represents reference material only. It is not intended as a medical manual, and the data presented here is meant to assist the reader in making informed choices regarding wellness. This book is not a replacement for treatment(s) that may have been suggested by the reader's personal physician. If the reader believes he or she is experiencing a medical issue, professional medical help is recommended. Mention of particular products, companies, or authorities in this book does not entail endorsement by the publisher or author.

INTRODUCTION

Aging is an inevitable part of life, and as we age, our brains change. The way they change, however, can be influenced by numerous factors. While we are small children, the goal of our parents and teachers is to provide us with enriched, stimulating environments to facilitate the greatest possible chance of developing normally, or in some cases even exceptionally. "Exceptional" here is not in regard to above average performance, but rather refers to individuals who begin life with a disability. For example, children who experience a developmental disadvantage or disability may have the opportunity to participate in programs that give these children the potential to achieve "for them" above average cognitive ability. But, you might ask, what happens if I am fifty-five, sixty-five, seventy-five, eighty-five, or ninety years old or older? Is there any advantage to putting into place a program to enrich my cognitive ability? This is the issue we will address and examine in this book.

Society's concern with brain development and, more specifically, with brain maintenance has significantly increased in recent years; the evidence shows that individuals are living substantially longer lives than previous generations. Historically, however, the focus has been on early brain development, and there is a clear lack of information for individuals who want to age successfully and aspire to maintain a high quality of life. This book presents evidentiary information on the best ways to ensure good cognitive ability as you age. Topics such as cognitive training, exercise, and diet, and how these all affect one's aging brain, will also be reviewed. It is important to understand that ensuring brain health as you age will require you to be proactive and to understand when things become abnormal. This book will give you insight into how the brain changes as we age and will explain what this means, and what you can do to help maintain effective cognitive ability. There are many products and strategies offering ways to maintain a youthful brain, but keep in mind that a youthful brain can be at a disadvantage compared to an experienced brain. Thus, the goal should not be achieving a youthful brain—we have worked hard to get to this point and do not want to regress; we want to progress. Therefore, the key should be to maintain our effective cognitive abilities as we reach our latter years. The information provided is intended to help you understand ways this can be achieved and to provide solid evidence of why things work the way they work and what you can do to minimize the effects of advancing age and combat certain diseases affecting the brain.

The brain has historically been divided into four major anatomical lobes; each of these lobes is believed to operate specific behavioral and sensory functions. The first few chapters will outline the major function of each lobe and provide insight into ways to stimulate these regions. The overall goal is to stimulate as much of the brain as possible to maintain brain health.

These four regions, or lobes, are called the frontal, parietal, temporal, and occipital. Each of these areas "contains" specific features involved in our everyday functioning. How we interact with the external world is driven by internal processes; specifically, the flow of information from our brain provides meaning and structure, and generates appropriate actions. It is important to note that at this point, even though we can discuss the regional components of the brain as if they are distinct, I do not believe that the brain works in a compartmental way. In fact, the different areas of the brain are connected in ways we are only beginning to understand. I will touch more on brain connectivity and neuroplasticity in the final chapter, but to begin this book I will discuss the processes involved in each of the identified brain regions, including a brief review of each area. These reviews will include a description of how functioning is evaluated, the effects of aging, and strategies to enhance cognitive ability using very simple tasks.

As we age, we are more susceptible to certain diseases affecting the brain; some can significantly impact one's quality of life. Although there are many diseases that can affect the brain, I have focused on one of the most debilitating neurodegenerative diseases linked to aging: Alzheimer's disease (AD). In addition, I will focus on one of the most common precursor illnesses linked to AD that is also of great concern, mild cognitive impairment (MCI). AD is a destroyer of cognitive ability, and it profoundly affects cognitive performance and a sense of oneself in everyone it touches. It is one of the most concerning issues of our global aging population. The section on AD includes pertinent information on ways you can fight the onset and progression of AD, as well as insight into factors related to living with AD.

This book strives to provide detailed and concise information on current research as well as information on how to stave off the onset of AD as much as possible. I provide the reader with succinct information about current medications commonly associated with treating AD and the role of medications in effectively managing the disease. I also provide general information on ways individuals can, and should, advocate for effective health care to fight this illness as soon as possible, and in the best ways possible.

The last two sections of the book focus on how to ensure healthy living and a healthy brain as you age. Understanding current information and evidence on the brain-aging process will go a long way to helping you put into place a program and lifestyle that can be neuroprotective to ensure successful brain aging. The final chapter examines the possible directions and avenues science may take in the years to come in regard to altering the effects of aging. Only by posing interesting questions will individuals be inspired to understand and answer them; thus I will provide some theories and examine the possibility of having excellent brain health forever. This will include looking at some of the scientific advancements that could make this possible. A glimpse into the future of what might be possible may help generate and spark ideas to deal with the issues we are all currently facing as we age.

Finally, the ultimate goal of this book is to provide proper and supportive information as both a resource tool and an instructional manual to inspire you to choose a path to good cognitive health as you age, and demonstrate why and how it is possible.

Section I

Cognitive Stimulation

I

THE BRAIN AGE

As our global village grows, so does our desire and expectation to access information instantly. With this growth of the technological age and the dawn of this new "instant information society," our ability to measure our personal performance both physically and mentally has become very accessible. For example, if we want to track how far we run or walk, we now can use a personal global position device (pGPS), which can also continuously monitor our heart rate, speed, pace, and so on. To top it off, we can have all this information instantly and remotely downloaded onto a computer as soon as we walk in our front door. These results can be ready in minutes and printed, or remotely reviewed, by whoever has access to this program. Thus, technology has reached a point where understanding physiologically how one is performing during a certain activity, and sharing this information widely, has been altered by how we access, store, and transmit personal information.

In regard to examining one's cognitive ability, there are certainly ways one can get a measure of basic ability. For example, there are several computer programs and websites that will test cognitive abilities in several areas (e.g., memory, vocabulary, perception). In addition to tests of cognitive performance, there are also commercially available programs that can track patterns of brain activation while performing cognitive tasks. With advancements over the next few decades, having an individual perform a task while their brain activation patterns are monitored remotely might soon be possible.

For example, in the field of genetics, scientists can now sequence people's entire genomes, which can help identify any diseases an individual may be predisposed to. These types of advances were thought unattainable even two decades ago. Similar to gene sequencing advances, neuroimaging advances can, to a certain extent, examine brain activation patterns for use in understanding an individual's predispositions to certain functional/cognitive deficits or the presence of or predisposition toward diseases. In addition, it is also not too far-fetched to think that in the future monitoring brain patterns while people are working on day-to-day activities could determine, for example, which times of day seem most productive, or at what times one should take a break, or when an individual might be in a state that makes them more susceptible to mistakes. Identifying physiological issues before the individual is consciously able to understand his or her limitations could be extremely important. I am certain you can think of many occupations that could benefit from this kind of technology (e.g., airline pilots, air traffic controllers, surgeons). The point is that there is a vast amount to be learned about the brain and, specifically, about the aging and adult brain. This is more important than ever before because life expectancy has significantly increased, and humans are living approximately twice as long as they did a century ago. The aging brain is, in some ways, a very new concern of the twenty-first century; understanding how to manage brain issues related to aging, and not just aging concerns related to one's physical abilities, is becoming an (anxious) issue for many. The emergence of this older and aging brain can be thought of, in some cases, as an unexplored frontier. Trying to understand the role played by eighty-six billion neurons (roughly fourteen billion fewer than is popularly suggested)[1] as one's age increases, as well as the creating and maintaining of successful neural connections throughout the aging process, will be a monumental and novel task to say the very least. Though the task is large, there are increasing numbers of neuroscientists working on understanding the role of the brain in almost every area one can think of, and schools are now specifically graduating neuroscientists whose whole focus is understanding the brain's inner workings, including functions, abilities, limitations, and so on. Thus, when I suggest that we are living in a "brain age," I mean we are living in an age in which understanding how the brain functions and responds in the face of so many events is at the forefront of the consciousness of society as a whole, and it seems to seep into our days in ways that many individuals may not be aware of. This process has inspired a new wave of researchers and a thirst for understanding more and more of what our brain's abilities, or limitations, are. As the global society ages, finding ways to maintain one's cognitive performance will drive research dollars and subsequently research programs, which will seek to answer how one can maintain a healthy brain and good cognitive performance into old age.

In the spirit of this brain age, I will review a couple of topics describing how this new focus on brain health has shaped our current research interests. Though it is essential to understand the pitfalls associated with aging, it is equally important to highlight positive aspects of aging and how aging may not affect one as expected. First off, I will describe the story of "SuperAgers" and how research shows that these individuals' brains do not act their age.[2] Second, I will review research examining aspects of aging and technology, specially looking at what is being developed to support aging individuals and how these new tools will change our future.

EXCEPTIONAL BRAIN AGING

Though time (aging) is detrimental for so many physiological processes, including the brain, it is not always so. In fact, researchers have documented subgroups of aging individuals that go against the conventional knowledge that aging equals "reduced brain ability." These individuals have been effectively identified as "SuperAgers."[3] Historically, there is an accepted understanding that as one ages one can expect to experience a decline or a significant reduction in cognitive ability. But this is not necessarily the case, and some individuals actually maintain excellent cognitive performance throughout their later years. When questioned, many individuals believe that aging equals a significant decline in cognitive ability. You might hear someone say, "I am having a seniors' moment." For some, this could actually be a positive experience, if they are one of these SuperAgers, and not the negative episode some intend by this statement.

The SuperAgers study focused on twelve individuals with an average age of 83.5, plus or minus 3 years. These individuals were compared to ten individuals of a similar age—83.1, plus or minus 3.4 years—and fourteen middle-aged individuals with an average age of 57.9, plus or minus 4.3 years. All individuals were tested on a range of memory-related tests, and their brains were measured via structural magnetic resonance imaging (MRI) to determine the level of cortical thickness for each group. Interestingly, the SuperAgers performed at a similar level as the middle-aged individuals on tests related to episodic memory (e.g., memory of life events, times, and places) and significantly better than others their age. What was even more remarkable was that when researchers measured whole-brain cortical thickness (brain size), they discovered that the SuperAgers displayed a similar level of cortical thickness as the middle-aged individuals, who were on average almost thirty years younger. This is remarkable because, typically, as individuals age their brains will often lose cortical thickness (reduce in size); in fact, the additional ten individuals with an average age of 83.1 showed a reduction of cortical thickness. The first assumption one might make is that these SuperAgers always had superior memories, in addition to significant education levels. However, the researchers noted that the SuperAgers were not noted to have superior skills when they were younger, and only four of the twelve had a university or college degree.[4]

This leaves a lot of unanswered questions related to how these individuals maintained this biological and cognitive advantage. Though how this was accomplished is certainly important, what might be more crucial is that it was actually achievable. As an eighty-year-old, it would certainly be quite beneficial to be a SuperAger, and it is not as unbelievable as one might have previously imaged. Thus, even before we get into the heart of this book, note that it is certainly possible to maintain cognitive ability as you age, and one should not expect, or accept, a loss of cognitive abilities with advancing age. The strategies outlined throughout this book are designed to put readers on the right track and give them the best opportunity to become one of these SuperAgers.

AGING AND TECHNOLOGY

For some individuals, the ability to maintain excellent cognitive performance may not be a real option, for any number of reasons (e.g., injury, disease). However, with this ever-evolving technological age we live in, we have developed electronic solutions in cases where the brain may fail to perform at our desired standards. The real challenge for many developers and designers has been to provide user-friendly systems for aging individuals. One might think that older individuals have an opposition to learning and understanding computer-assisted devices or new technology in general. However, research suggests that this is just not the case, and that older people are not "technophobic" and are more receptive to learning new technologies than traditionally thought.[5] The key to successful implementation of good electronic and computerized assisted devices for older individuals is ensuring that they are used effectively. It is also suggested that older individuals should be provided with extra training time to learn how to use these devices to their best advantage. As well, these devices need to be as user-friendly as possible, starting with a clear and effective menu that defines the features of the equipment well.

The devices potentially available to support aging individuals seem only limited by our imagination. One of the most interesting devices, encompassing many smaller integrated devices, is "smart home" technology. The stated role of the smart home is to ensure safety and independence for the resident.[6] The smart home can include technology that monitors the stability of the resident by using sensors installed throughout the home to determine if the individual has, for example, fallen to the ground. Basic features can also include automatic lighting, which lights the room as the individual enters, or voice-activated TV or radio. Other features can be more sophisticated, such as motion sensors to track the individual's activities throughout the day. This feature can provide caregivers with daily feedback on how much time the individual spent in different areas of the home. For example, tracking the amount of time spent in the kitchen could suggest whether or not meals were prepared and consumed. Moreover, smart homes can integrate technology such as wearable body sensors or items such as a bio-sensing shirts, which have the ability to detect and continuously track an individual's biorhythms (e.g., heart rate). Sensor development has progressed to the extent that they can be placed directly on clothing and linked, for example, to one's washing machine; individuals can put their wash in the machine, and it will automatically determine which type of wash cycle to perform. Another great feature of the smart home is that systems can be operated through a touch screen menu. Thus, with clear menu icons that easily identify various features of the house, users can, for example, see who is at the front door or open and close doors, windows, and blinds. Smart homes can also be equipped with technology that will help the individual maintain their routine. For instance, if an individual isn't sure what to do next at any time during the day, they can query "the home" via a voice-activated system and ask what the next task they normally perform is on this day of the week. Individuals can also ask the home what time they can expect their caregiver and how many minutes are left until their arrival. This feature is especially important for individuals with a cognitive impairment; having the ability to ask questions without worrying about ridicule or without frustrating a caregiver can be of great use. In addition, if an individual with a cognitive impairment is left at home alone, they can query the smart home for answers to questions over and over again, eliminating much of the frustration and anxiety an individual can experience when they become unsure of something. A caregiver can also program in suggested activities for the individual while they are away, which can include automatic reminders. Built-in features can also include automatic voice reminders of appointments or scheduled phone calls. Smart homes can also be used to program medication dispensing, which can utilize face-recognition systems so that if there are a few individuals in the home the proper type and dose of medication is delivered to the proper person. Automatic systems for locking the doors or turning off the bath water or the stove have also been identified as standard smart home technology inclusions. The real benefit to having a system like this in place is that it can reduce fears associated with living alone or with an aging significant other. The goal of these homes is to ensure greater quality of life for individuals so they can age in place. Incurring a drastic change in one's quality of life (e.g., leaving the family home) can cause a significant amount of stress; if a situation arises where the individual may not be safe at home, the technology presented here could certainly increase the opportunities for individuals to maintain their independence and their comfortable home environment.[7]

In addition to these features of the smart home, other researchers have suggested that there can be great benefits to using computers for two-way video use. Having a computer available and accessible so an individual can accept or decline video calls or be set up for daily check-ins with family or caregivers is an excellent way for an individual to maintain positive relationships.[8] These types of systems can also be used by health-care professionals to see and talk to the individual and readily determine needs in situations where this might have otherwise been very difficult. These types of video assessments have risen in use and implementation, particularly in regions where accessing the individual due to geography can be difficult (e.g., long travel distances or inaccessible towns).[9] These types of interactive systems may also be very helpful in situations where overburdened clinics need to track an individual's health. Thus, a virtual appointment might occur much sooner than an in-person one, and at limited cost.

For many aging individuals, having a virtual appointment or a virtual chat with family will certainly pale in comparison to a real visit. However, in some cases, when used effectively and individuals are aware of the facts and the feelings of all involved (not ideal in some cases), these types of systems can be used in a positive fashion to ensure that connections are maintained and regular in-person visits are richer. Individuals are provided the opportunity to feel more in touch with the happenings in each other's lives. The key is certainly ensuring that this type of interaction does not replace in-person contact but is instead used to enhance relationships. For many aging individuals, the future will include an increase in video interactions, which can be a great way for an aging parent to check in with their family and for families to check in with an aging parent.

As one can see, in-home applications of technology have certainly come a long way in the last decade. These advantages, however, have not stopped at the development of in-home devices. Unlike previous generations, we are a very mobile global society; because we are so mobile, technology has had to keep pace and integrate with our needs and wants. So-called smart phones use a significant amount of specialized technology, including global positioning systems (GPS). The inclusion of GPS allows individuals access to a map that can determine their location and provide step-by-step instructions on how to reach a desired destination. These smart phones also double as a personal assistant, providing one the ability to input dates into a calendar and ensure that reminders are given prior to appointment times. These phones can also be used to make notes or write down a grocery list, check online for better deals when at a store, and stay in touch via text message or e-mail at any given time. Smart phones can also act as a virtual wallet, allowing one to pay for items with the phone. Individuals can also closely track their bank accounts, including daily and monthly transactions, and be alerted of any concerns. Effectively, the smart phone becomes an electronic personal banker as well.

A lingering question many aging individuals have is, "If I rely heavily on this technology, am I not compromising brain ability because I will not be using my mind as much?" This is a great question, and a great fear of many aging individuals, and rightly so. However, researchers have suggested that using technology effectively actually involves a significant amount of brain resources. For example, inputting dates and reminders into your calendar requires both brain activation and cognitive involvement in scheduling weekly or monthly tasks. Asking for directions, be it from your smart phone or in person, requires one to dedicate cognitive resources. In fact, inputting directional information into your smart phone requires activating the visual and motor cortices networks (beyond what would be experienced via verbal directions). In addition, these phones can be used to track and improve our eating habits and exercise levels, both of which will be shown in this book to be very important for brain health as we age. These phones also allow us to maintain social connections beyond what has been previously available.[10] To some aging individuals, all this knowledge about what capabilities phones like these possess can be very daunting. Things like updating software and downloading programs will require time and brain effort that may not have been otherwise utilized. As you can see, a significant amount of brain resources will be required for these applications. Because this technology is ever emerging on the market, much of this will be quite novel to many aging individuals, especially in the next few years, and will require time and effort to learn the ins and outs of this equipment. Understanding and using these resources to the best of your ability will take time and significant mental effort, which might be just what your brain needs. Devices that require one to stay involved and be actively aware of needed changes or upgrades require one to relearn something new every now and then, which is an excellent way to keep one's brain engaged.

One might believe that these applications are only beneficial if one is a cognitively healthy aging individual, and if an individual has some memory issues already, then learning the technology related to a smart phone might be too difficult and unhelpful. Surprisingly, however, that has not been shown to be true. In fact, researchers have reported that individuals with moderate to severe memory issues have had good success (with training) in using commercially available programs for day-to-day memory tasks. Thus, not only were improvements seen, but researchers also showed that individuals with cognitive issues could be trained to use a smart phone to supplement memory concerns, thus closing the gap between themselves and cognitively intact individuals and creating greater independence, which is an excellent positive outcome for individuals who might previously have been very frustrated. [11]

As one can see, there are numerous technological advances coming each year, and creating an opportunity for aging individuals to use this technology to their advantage will be important for the aging society. It is important to highlight that, as with any new tool, with no prior experience individuals will require a certain amount of training time to master the skills involved, but once achieved the benefits can be great. Aging is currently a certainty for all individuals; however, how you age and at what rate is optional. The brain age is upon us. How we respond to the wealth of information that will be available to us over the next few years will certainly help shape our aging society's future. Thus, it is imperative for individuals who want good brain health, and to cognitively age well, to seek out and implement the best ways to do this. The remainder of this book is a collection of supported strategies and information to ensure that you are on the right track when it comes to ensuring good brain health.

2

WHAT DOES THE FRONT OF MY BRAIN DO AND WHY IS IT IMPORTANT AS I AGE?

After reading this chapter, you should be able to answer the following questions:

What kind of tasks does my frontal lobe perform?

How do researchers determine if the front of my brain is performing normally?

Does my frontal lobe have the ability to compensate for deficits in other areas of my brain?

Are there any activities I can perform to specifically activate my frontal cortex, and if so would it be beneficial for me to perform them?

The frontal lobe (figure 2.1) is known to be involved in a number of processes. It primarily directs our ability to organize activities, maintain attention, monitor progress, and act in a flexible manner. In addition, perseverance, perception, cognition (i.e., abstract reasoning), and certain sensory functions are just some of the other important features that areas within the frontal lobe perform. The initiation of these high-level activities often occurs primarily in this lobe, and as such it is often identified as the "executive center" because it provides structure and organization to the majority of tasks we perform each day.

Testing the functioning of our frontal lobe can occur in many ways. One of the least invasive ways is through neuropsychological evaluation. Using this method, researchers may, for instance, have individuals en-

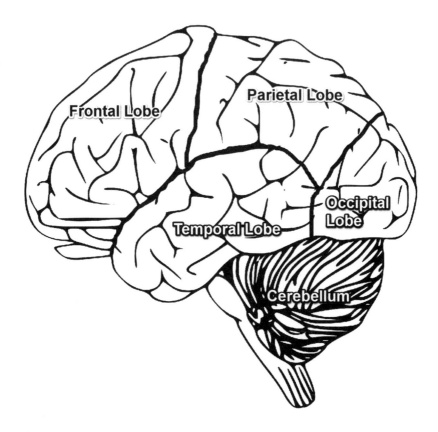

Figure 2.1. *Major Brain Lobes and the Cerebellum.* **This figure displays the location of the traditionally defined four major lobes of the brain and the cerebellum as viewed from the left side of the brain. (WJ Tippett/***Building an Ageless Mind.***Rowman & Littlefield Publishers, Inc.)**

gage in tasks that involve planning, foresight, or procedures requiring original thought, such as generating novel word lists. These types of tests are sensitive to neural disruptions that may occur as a result of damage to the frontal lobe. Thus, we know that neural disruptions to a certain extent can be detected via a simple paper-and-pencil procedure. One of the primary ways to detect neural distress or interference in the frontal lobe is through the presentation of neural incongruent tasks. What does this mean? Well, for example, if one is shown the word *blue* written in red ink and is asked to name the color of ink and not read the word, that would be an example of a neural incongruence task. This is an actual psychological task called the Stroop test; it has been used since the 1930s. What is interesting about the Stroop test is that the brain, and more specifically the anterior cingulate and dorsolateral prefrontal cortex[1] located in the frontal lobe, will process much of this information. When one is requested to answer these questions quickly, one must of course disregard the unimportant information and organize the correct information to generate the response needed, which in this example is "red." Tests such as these are very good measures of frontal lobe functioning. Though these tests have been used for quite some time, it was not until recently (in the last twenty-five years or so) that we have actually had the ability to (somewhat) look inside the brain while it is working to see where processing for tasks of this type occurs. Up until this time, researchers relied on studying individuals with specified brain damage to help determine what certain parts of the brain are used for and what deficits we can expect when damage occurs to these areas. However, these evaluations were limited in that detailed information of the precise brain areas that were being affected was hard to come by. As well, because patients' responses to injuries are so varied, researchers would have to use a composite of behavioral information from various individuals to get a general understanding of which structures, for example, in the frontal lobe, are responsible for planning a movement. With the introduction of imaging technology, specifically functional magnetic resonance imaging (fMRI), we now have a better idea of the areas of the brain that are at work during task performance. What fMRI measures is blood-oxygen level dependence (BOLD); basically, it examines the amount of oxygen used in the brain. Which area needs more O_2, researchers suggest, indicates greater activity and the region most likely responsible for task performance. In addition, much early research went to linking behavioral deficits in patients who had experienced trauma to certain brain regions to provide further evidence for regionalization of specific behavioral tasks to certain brain structures. Thus, it could be suggested that the best explanation for regionalization of specific tasks would be from these two lines of research, which form our current general understanding of what might be happening in the brain.

IMAGING RESEARCH AND THE FRONTAL LOBE

Conducting a scan of the brain (i.e., imaging) while it is at "rest" or at "work" (as with an fMRI) provides a new way to test which tasks are linked to which part of the brain. Another advantage is that researchers are able to make comparisons between individuals of varying ages to determine how the brain changes and operates differently as we age.

The multitude of imaging studies available demonstrates that the frontal lobe is significantly involved in activities such as the processing of novel words,[2] indicating that new information needs to be attended to, and acted on, in a meaningful manner to be useful at a later time. Additional research has noted that the frontal region contains very fine distinctions; although the brain generally operates in collusion, damage to general areas of the right frontal, left frontal, or bifrontal regions produces very different types of cognitive deficits. These deficits can affect, for example, one's ability to process phonemic (segments of sounds in a word) fluency[3] or one's ability to organize information for the purpose of remembering, generally noted as a prefrontal cortex task.[4] The frontal lobe has also been noted as central to our ability to comprehend language,[5] understand word meaning,[6] and reason effectively[7]; the list of these higher-level processing tasks goes on and on. The primary point I am trying to make is that this region is essential to effectively interact with the external world and apply meaning and organization to the information we are faced with on a daily basis. It is also important to note that our frontal lobe is the region that helps us, as humans, form the concept of self and self-awareness. Patients experiencing frontotemporal dementia (FTD) often lose their concept of self or self-awareness.[8] Individuals can have great difficulty acting in their own self-interest and even demonstrate a lack of understanding of the level of their own deficit. These individuals often have difficulty managing their own finances (similar to Alzheimer's disease [AD] patients) and are reported to show signs of disinhibition related to social conventions (for example, dressing appropriately in public) and can act in an inappropriate sexual manner to individuals of the opposite sex. These individuals may also experience a disinterest in tasks once deemed enjoyable or engage in other tasks they once thought silly.

Thus, the concept of who they were or are as a person can start to deteriorate. Since a disease like FTD can have dramatic effects on an individual's understanding of self, I will discuss FTD before reviewing brain changes as we age.

FRONTOTEMPORAL DEMENTIA

FTD is a term used to define individuals that demonstrate identified brain atrophy (e.g., dementia) in the frontal and temporal regions. Researchers historically have also used *Pick's disease* interchangeably with FTD, but more recently FTD and its subdesignation frontal variant frontal temporal dementia (FvFTD) seem to be the common designations for the pathological effects observed in the frontal regions of the brain. FTD is currently thought to come about because of a gene mutation involving chromosome 17, which involves the production of neurofibrillary tangles. These occur when the internal structure of a cell begins to break down due to the accumulation of an abnormal protein called tau, causing a breakdown in the cell's system to feed itself, which kills the brain cell from the inside out.[9] The frontal lobe of the brain is commonly considered the "executive center" of the brain. Many daily activities we perform, such as planning, organizing, social conduct/ awareness, mood, name finding, and many other higher-level behavioral activities are thought to be the primary responsibility of the frontal regions. With this in mind, many researchers believe that identifying individuals with FTD should not be difficult because there are readily identifiable behavioral deficits that stand out in contrast to individuals with AD. However, as you might imagine, using behavioral measures on both of these types of populations might be easier said than done. Many deficits arising out of each disease are very similar. Thus, unless you have access to a clinic that has well-identified procedures to distinguish between these diseases, including access to imaging data, an individual will most likely be diagnosed with AD or a dementia-related illness. Conversely, individuals who present with "typical" frontal lobe difficulties, and are on average younger than many individuals with AD, may receive a FTD diagnosis initially, until further investigated.

There has been some research trying to find reliable behavioral criteria to discriminate between AD and FTD individuals. Though a 100 percent reliability cannot be found, the following traits are some of the ones primarily noted as good discriminative factors between these groups. For example, research comparing AD against FvFTD patients has noted significant differences on tasks such as attention, visual perception, constructive praxis (problems drawing or copying figures), and memory (specifically the ability to complete short story recall and reconstructing figures from memory given a short delay period).[10] FvFTD patients have also been shown to be different from AD patients because of their lack of social awareness, stereotypical movements (a pattern or fixed behavioral movements), and eating habits,[11] which occurred regardless of how severely individuals were affected by the disease. Finally, another main difference between AD and FvFTD patients is in their ability to infer what other individuals' thoughts, feelings, and mental states were given a certain social situation. Mild FvFTD individuals were noted to have problems understanding what other individuals might be experiencing; their abilities were similar to how children between the ages of three and seven perform on certain social tests.[12] As can be seen, having insight and inference into others' states of mind can be significantly impaired for FTD patients, but not AD patients.

Surprisingly, researchers have demonstrated that factors such as mood changes, executive dysfunction, and self-care,[13] as well as linguistic, executive, and intellective abilities,[14] were not good discriminators between individuals with AD and FvFTD. These results are unexpected in that many of these traits are highlighted as major reasons for providing an FTD versus an AD diagnosis. Additionally, much of the research to date has suffered from low recruitment numbers, which most certainly would contribute to the difficulty of identifying the key aspects of FTD versus AD. Because these differences can sometimes be subtle, especially in certain cases, it makes it almost impossible to untangle which group the individual should belong to. As well, it is important to remember that individuals react differently to each disease, which again makes it difficult to accurately diagnose, particularly because there can be so many overlapping features/symptoms. Researchers and clinicians, therefore, do the best they can with the tools they have and the information available to them at the time. I think the best advice is to be proactive and read up on the subtle differences between AD and FTD. Reporting and tracking all the symptoms an individual experiences can make a big difference in how he or she is diagnosed, which may have a dramatic effect on his or her care plan.

Finally, it is important to point out that an illness such as FTD can have dramatic effects on who a person is. As shown, the frontal lobe is an essential region to ensure normal functioning. Because of the significant responsibility of the frontal regions in our everyday performance, it is important to understand how it changes and how it is affected as one ages.

BRAIN CHANGES AS WE AGE

Before moving into the brain training section of this chapter, it is important to examine some of the observable changes that occur in the frontal lobe of the brain as we age. Most studies examining older individuals have indicated that better cognitive performance is correlated to increased brain activity. In addition, the frontal cortex is the one region that is often found to have increased activity as we age.[15] One reason this increase is occurring is that the frontal cortex may be acting as a compensatory system,[16] filling in for other regional deficiencies in an effort to maintain "regular" performance and to ensure activities or tasks can be produced in a timely and efficient manner. What is not known is the extent of this process. Does every aging individual have this inborn capacity? Are some individuals better at it than others? Do they experience success each and every time they draw on these additional resources? These are questions researchers do not have the answers to yet, but I am confident these issues will be studied and broached in the near future. What I can tell you is that accessing additional resources within the frontal lobe to help individuals function at an optimal level is a good argument for brain training and theories related to brain plasticity. Engaging in tasks that activate regions in the frontal lobe on a regular basis could greatly benefit cognition and brain function. Hence, one of the primary roles of this book is to provide individuals with simple ways to increase brain activation in specific regions, and subsequently increase cognitive performance as we age. Provided below are a few simple activities one can perform to help activate his or her frontal cortex. In addition, I have provided simple ways you can, on your own, change these tasks to keep them fresh and novel as you move forward, which as you will see later in this book is essential for brain health.

TRAINING THE FRONTAL LOBE

One of the primary features of the brain's frontal region is its ability to cognitively control ongoing events. Research has shown that the frontal lobe can be further segregated when humans are performing specified tasks. For example, an area within the frontal lobe known as the dorsolateral prefrontal cortex (DLPFC) (see figure 2.2) is linked to our ability to hold information "online" in order to complete the entire steps of a specified procedure. Also, this area can, if required, modify task performance to change the direction or duration of specified tasks as needed. The DLPFC is tied to our attention system, and it provides us, as humans, the ability to attend to tasks at hand.

The idea that the frontal lobe is the brain's control center has not been lost on several researchers. Some of the most cutting-edge research has involved using the brain as a system to control our external world via a human-computer interface system. An example of how this has been achieved is through the implantation of electrical devices to interact with the brain. In fact, implantation of devices into the frontal region has been used to help individuals with limited or no mobility operate items such as the lights in their room, the television, the curtains, and so on.[17] These types of advances demonstrate the control our frontal lobe has over our actions, and in some cases our external environment. We know that engaging in tasks similar to the ones noted in the opening of this chapter will activate the frontal lobe. We also know through electroencephalography (EEG) and fMRI research that the more this area is activated, the more efficiently it processes information of this nature, and the more "automatic" the process becomes.

This evidence is important because continued training and repetitive activation of independent regions may keep these areas healthier longer and help stave off brain diseases such as AD and may also provide quicker recovery if one is affected by a traumatic event, such as a traumatic brain injury or a stroke. It is also important to note that little information is provided to aging individuals in regard to the maintenance of brain regions. But to maintain a healthy brain, one needs to partake in activities that stimulate all brain regions; in particular, one should take time to active each brain region specifically. Thus, in the following section, suggestions are provided for activities one can do to activate and stimulate the frontal lobe.

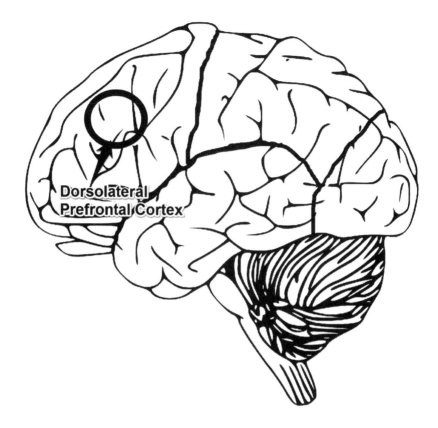

Figure 2.2.   *The Dorsolateral Prefrontal Cortex (DLPFC).* The approximate location
(left side of the brain) of the **DLPFC** within the frontal lobe. **(WJ Tippett/***Building
an Ageless Mind.* **Rowman & Littlefield Publishers, Inc.)**

FRONTAL LOBE ACTIVITIES

As humans, we live in a rule-based society where one action results in
the occurrence of a secondary action. The majority of the time we are
operating from the position of experience, and as such we often have
preconceived expectations of what may occur. For example, if I throw a
rock at a window, I expect the window will break, but I do not wonder if
the rock will fly through the air because I know that the laws of physics
dictate that the rock will fly. What is left to determine are variables such
as distance, height, flight time, and so on. I provide this simplistic example to point out that individuals with healthy brains take many things
that seem rather simple for granted; when things do not work the way

one would expect them to, it is accompanied by a significant amount of distress and frustration. Thus, if you are an individual afflicted with a cognitive impairment, this frustration and distress becomes a part of your everyday life. For instance, the action of picking up a rock and throwing it is one that requires integration and communication between various areas of the brain. A healthy brain is required to ensure that one can complete a multitude of procedural steps in order to carry out a specified action in a unified manner (both internally and externally), each and every minute of every day. Keeping the brain "flexible" and healthy should be an essential component for us all; this could help us deal with aging and disease. Let me provide a quick example of our brains' expectations. The next time you turn on your computer, before using your mouse, pick it up and turn it sideways. Now try to use it as you would normally (e.g., same hand placement) and pick a point on the screen you would like your cursor to touch. What you will find is that it is no longer as simple a task as it normally is, and it requires a "remapping" of sorts to allow you to complete it correctly. This is because our brain has been wired to operate this way, based on our preconditioned experience. The point is that because of these everyday expectations few cerebral challenges are thrust in our path; to keep an active and healthy brain, we need to participate in tasks that are challenging and ever changing.

Here are a few activities that I have come up with that you can use to challenge yourself. These activities are specifically designed to activate your frontal lobe.

Activity One—Processing

Activity One Instructions: On the left side you will see a column of numbers and a column indicating which hand you will be required to use (e.g., left, right, or both). On the right side you will see four sets of circles with the numbers 1 or 2 above them. For the first time through, you will use the hand indicated and touch the target as indicated. For example, for the first one you will take your left hand and touch the left side of target number 1; for the third one you will take your right hand and touch target 1 on the right side. Make sure you pick a starting location below the page for both hands and use this location to begin and end the task with.

1. The first time through you will do exactly as indicated.
2. The second time through use the opposite hand. For example, on task 1 you would now use your right hand instead of your left, and you must remember this rule throughout the second time through (note: for both hands you will still use both hands).
3. For the third time through, you will use the opposite number. For instance, on task 1 you will use the left hand as indicated but touch target number 2 instead of target number 1.
4. Finally, for the fourth time through, you will use the opposite hand and the opposite number. For example, for task 1 you would use your right hand to touch the target on the right side marked target number 2, not target number 1.

Repeat this task five times. Record your times to see if you become faster.

If you start to see good improvement, modify the task on your own by changing the order of the hand used or the number used or both. Track your progress on each procedure type (i.e., each modification you make) to see if you improve and make changes accordingly. This will ensure an ever-changing and challenging procedure you can modify on your own.

Table 2.1.   Targets

1-Left		
2-Left		
1-Right	2	2
2-Both	O	O
1-Left		
2-Right	1	1
1-Both	O	O
2-Left		
1-Right		

Activity Two—Ordering

Activity Two Instructions: On day one you will write out the alphabet and give each letter a corresponding number, skipping every second letter and every second number. For example, A = 1, C = 3, E = 5, and so on. Then you will go back and fill in the skipped numbers: for example, B = 2, D = 4, and so on. This will create two rows, one with odd numbers and letters and one with even numbers and letters (see below). With the corresponding letters and numbers spell words numerically.

A-1, C-3, E-5, G-7, I-9, K-11, M-13, O-15, Q-17, S-19, U-21, W-23, Y-25

B-2, D-4, F-6, H-8, J-10, L-12, N-14, P-16, R-18, T-20, V-22, X-24, Z-26

For example, try spelling the word *brain* numerically: 2, 18, 1, 9, 14 = 44.

Now try the words *health, exercise, connections, stimulate*. Time yourself and see how well you did by both completion time and the number of words added correctly. Once you get sufficiently good at this task, *change it*.

Instead, write the alphabet out starting with the letter *B* and the number *1*, skipping each letter and each number, creating a new row of numbers and letters ending with the letter *A*. Create a new word list (five or ten words or as many as you want), and spell them out numerically, add them together, and see how well you did. Repeat each day until you get good at this task and then *change it again*.

Activity Three—Free Word Association

Activity Three Instructions: Pick two letters of the alphabet. For example, the letter *A* and the letter *T*. Give yourself ninety seconds to name as many things as you can think of that one would find in a grocery store that begins with the letter *A* (write them down). Then try it again with the letter *T*. Next, name as many things as you can think of that you would find in a school that start with the letters *A* and *T*, remembering to time yourself and write down your answers. When you have completed the task, count how many words you were able to name each time. Repeat this each day until you see good improvement; once you do, change the two letters you were using. With your new letters, repeat this task again for a few days until you see improvement, and then *change your letters again.*

The role of these tasks is to enhance your brain through activities that stimulate your frontal lobe. The tasks designed, though rather simplistic, provide you with a starting point and the tools to modify and change them with little effort. Though the modifications are relatively simple, you will notice that great effort is required to adapt to the new tasks, which as you will learn, is the cornerstone to a healthy brain.

3

WHERE IT ALL COMES TOGETHER

The Parietal Lobe

After reading this chapter, you should be able to answer the following questions:

What is the role of the parietal lobe in completing visually guided
   movements?
Will aging affect my ability to make visually guided movements?
Are there any activities I can perform to specifically activate my
   parietal cortex, and if so would it be beneficial for me to perform
   them?

In the last chapter I suggested that you try turning your computer
mouse sideways before using it and see how effective you were at locating a desired point on the screen. For some people this task is extremely
difficult, while others take a short time to make the adjustment. You
may wonder why I am pointing this example out one more time; the
reason is that the area of the brain responsible for integrating incoming
visual information (where we see the cursor on the screen) to generate
a motor output (moving it to the desired position) is essentially the
responsibility of the parietal lobe. The parietal lobe/region (see figure
2.1) is the area of the brain primarily responsible for supporting visually
guided movements.

   As you can see from figure 2.1, the parietal lobe is an area that starts
approximately at the top of your head just before your head begins to

become round (hopefully) and from there extends to the back of the head and is about the width of your hand and a half. This part of your brain is a very exciting region in that it is responsible for performing many tasks we take for granted. For example, this region is involved in the control and direction of our eye movements (e.g., gaze, tracking objects). It is also linked directly to our ability to successfully perform reaching, pointing, and grasping activities, including the updating of ongoing motor plans. For instance, if we reach for a glass on a table and the table starts to shift and the glass begins to move, our parietal region (specifically, the posterior parietal cortex) will transform this visual information to update the location of the glass and create a motor plan to alter our reach and grab the glass before it falls off the table. Thus, eye-hand coordination is one of the primary features of this brain region.

The parietal lobe is our vision-for-action center and is one of the predominant ways that we interact with our external world. Using vision to guide motor responses is for many individuals an unconscious and seamless act. Every day the parietal lobe performs endless numbers of these acts that one would perceive are very simple. However, this process is a very complex one and requires the integration of numerous amounts of information that all primarily converge on the parietal lobe. This information must then be converted and sent on to the premotor and motor areas to produce an efficient and effective motor response. If this region (specifically the posterior parietal cortex) experiences trauma or damage, research has shown that individuals will experience difficulty programming visually guided eye and arm movements.[1]

It is important to state here that the parietal region does not work in isolation but constantly sends and receives information from both the frontal and medial-temporal (middle part of your brain, see figure 2.1) areas of the brain. In the example of reaching for a glass, grabbing the glass before it hits the ground not only requires several visuomotor (vision and motor) plans but may rely on our personal experiences, such as knowing that the table always falls to the right. With this knowledge provided by additional brain regions, we choose and carry out what we believe is the best response.

One of the primary ways researchers have tested the parietal lobe is through neuropsychological visuospatial tasks. The basics of these types of procedures normally require individuals to demonstrate intact abilities through the copying of complex designs, such as in the Rey-Osterrieth Complex Figure Test,[2] or to identify the relative spatial locations of arbitrary lines, as in the Benton Line Orientation Test.[3] Inability to complete these types of procedures or even to complete a simple task such as copying a picture of two overlaid pentagons crossing one another (investigators are looking for precision in such a simple task as this) indicates that something may not be right. Individuals' inability to perform these types of tasks may indicate to an investigator that the region of the brain responsible for these elements (which we now know is the parietal lobe) could be affected. It is also important to note that these tests are flexible enough that one should not be concerned that being a bad drawer will lead investigators to believe that there is something wrong. These tests are set up to detect real disturbances and deficits that are usually fairly obvious to a trained researcher. I should also point out that all neuropsychological evaluations are created to account for normal differences observed in the general population, such as education level, age, or sex of the participant. Each one of these attributes can influence how individuals perform; therefore, comparisons are made relative to a similar population. Though I have provided some examples of tasks that are performed within the parietal lobe, I would also like to highlight some recent imaging evidence to demonstrate how involved this region is in everyday tasks.

IMAGING RESEARCH AND THE PARIETAL LOBE

Imaging researchers have shown the parietal lobe to be involved in completing activities such as line bisection (detecting the midpoint of a line), visual motion, spatial realignment (correcting vision for action when experiencing distortions), visual search, goal directed hand movements, as well as the other activities I have already mentioned.[4] The take-home message from this research is that the parietal region is very important in completing and maintaining visually guided motor control. Without a functioning parietal cortex, performing everyday acts such as grabbing that glass of water would be very difficult, if not impossible. One of the questions researchers are interested in is how the area changes as we age. Should you expect significant reductions in your visual motor ability?

BRAIN CHANGES AS WE AGE

As I have previously discussed, as we age our brains change. In some cases, they change dramatically, while in other cases they progress at a steady rate. Either way, this process is constant. These changes, of course, are not readily observable, and as a result, you may wonder, "Will I still function at the level I have always been accustomed to as I reach my latter years?" This chapter focuses on the parietal lobe, and as such I will address how aging affects activities involving parietal lobe functioning.

The primary question with the parietal lobe is will aging affect your visually guided motor performance. Well, yes, of course it will. But the good news is that in most cases it is not that big of a change. Most interesting is that as we age our brain begins to operate somewhat differently than when we were younger. What is generally seen is that the older brain utilizes other brain regions to support task completion. Thus, activations become more widespread throughout the brain, unlike in younger brains where activations are more focused and are limited to specified regions.[5] This evidence indicates that older individuals must rely more on the whole brain for many activities we perform each day such as reaching and grasping, which is particularly important if the response required is extraordinary. But what you may really want to know is how this affects your performance. For basic reaching-type activities, research has shown that responses can be slowed by an average of 0.4 seconds.[6] However, if older individuals are given time to practice, this difference can become relatively small. This of course changes if the young individuals are given practice time as well, but nevertheless older individuals can perform relatively well.[7] So if you are planning to begin a career as a race car driver at sixty-five, you may want to rethink your decision, because half a second might make a big difference. But generally speaking, you should not see much of a degradation in your movement performance as it relates to the brain's ability.

A healthy brain as we age is important in supporting all types of activities beyond normally predefined regions. It is important to understand that other regions may rely on the parietal lobe to complete desired activities. For example, our working memory is vital to remembering things such as the page we were just reading, a phone number until we dial it, a message just after getting off the phone, and the like.

Though we know the brain region primarily responsible for this activity is the temporal lobe, researchers have shown that there is great reliance on the parietal lobe as well.[8] Additionally, current evidence examining the physiological structure of the nervous system via brain imaging examinations demonstrates that age-related declines in visual motor dexterity (e.g., dialing a phone number) and visuospatial construction (e.g., puzzle construction) can occur as a result of reduction in structural integrity in the inferior longitudinal fasciculus (a structure linking the parietal lobe to the frontal and temporal lobes).[9] Since we know that these regions can be weakened by age, trauma, or disease, activating this connective structure might provide the opposite response and strengthen these connections, helping overall brain health. Therefore, training the parietal lobe could be of great importance.

TRAINING THE PARIETAL LOBE

As I have outlined above, the parietal lobe is highly involved with everyday visually guided motor acts. This region includes areas that specialize in pointing, grasping, tracking of objects, updating our ongoing movements, navigating our external world, and basic calculations around how to successfully interact with items presented to us. Because we perform these acts day in and day out, one might think, "Why would I need to train this area; it is always at work?" This is an excellent point. However, though one would be correct in assuming that this area is always at work, these activities become very specialized and our brain gets so used to performing them that it expends little energy doing so, resulting in less brain activation. This is normally a very good thing in that little resources are being used to interact with our world and we can focus our attention and resources on more important things. If we constantly needed to focus on how to move about, we would be very frustrated and little else would be achieved during our day. The main point here is that the acts that we are performing do not challenge this region on a daily basis, and in a way the area can become complacent. For some, this may have become apparent, for instance, when trying a *new* activity that requires successful eye-hand coordination. Such an activity might have taken some time to get right. This is a good example of this region hard at work. The example of turning your computer mouse sideways is also a great demonstration of this area at work. It takes time to understand where and how to move your mouse, and these types of activities are excellent ways to exercise this region. With this in mind I have provided some example activities below that will stimulate and activate the parietal lobe and that I believe can assist in providing an overall healthy brain.

PARIETAL LOBE ACTIVITIES

Below I have again provided three suggested activities one can do to keep the parietal lobe stimulated and active. The first activity uses tangrams, puzzles that came from China and emerged in the Americas at the start of the 1800s. What I like about these puzzles is that they require the user to spatially understand and organize the location of pieces in a specific way to be successful. Thus, significant involvement of the parietal lobe can be expected, in both constantly manipulating the pieces as well as trying to work out how they should come together. The second activity is a 3-D puzzle construction. Again, this type of activity requires general spatial understanding and continued manipulation of the pieces, which will also assist in fine motor skill maintenance.

The final activity is a navigation one. This activity is physical and moves the user away from the table. It is important to point out that some researchers suggests that tabletop activities (such as paper-and-pencil tasks) can be independent of normal navigation ability, such as finding your way around streets or trails. Thus, individuals may actually perform satisfactorily on these measures, making the evaluation of true ability difficult to assess.[10] In fact, researchers have shown that some individuals can experience this specific deficit alone.[11] Thus, it is important to remember that if you see a brain training guide or package (e.g., a computer program or activity book) out in the market suggesting that this ability can be remediated using only paper-and-pencil activities, know that this may not in fact be the case. With this in mind, I have suggested actually performing a way-finding (navigation) training task using an environment you may be faced with every day (and if possible a novel environment).

Finally, I would like to point out that these again are example tasks that are designed to focus on stimulating the parietal lobe. There are, of course, any number of activities one could engage in to help keep this region active and challenged. I would like to suggest one other activity not included below, and that is the game *Pac-Man*. I really like *Pac-Man* as a training tool because the elements of the game require individuals to identify target positions, track moving objects, navigate a series of ever-changing virtual environments, and engage in avoidance maneuvers. These should all sound very familiar in that they require great involvement of the parietal lobe. In addition, as one gets better at it, the game becomes more challenging (i.e., faster ghosts, new game boards), which is excellent for creating an ongoing challenging activity for the user. There are a couple of ways you can get this game. One is by picking up a "plug-and-play" game console. These can be found at online stores or in special game stores (possibly even large department stores). These consoles include a joystick and two cables that plug directly into your TV, and nothing else is needed. Thus it does not require any significant set up, and you can plug it directly into any TV (approximate cost is anywhere from twenty to ninety dollars). The other way is to play online; there are a number of free sites that allow you to play online at your own computer. So, yes, believe it or not, I am suggesting you play some video games each week. After a while, you may even want to challenge your kids, grandkids, friends, significant other, or anyone else to game.

Activity One—Tangrams

A tangram puzzle consists of seven shapes: two small right triangles, two large right triangles, one medium right triangle, one parallelogram, and one square. I have provided a set of smaller tear-out pieces so you can try this task on your own and get a feel for manipulating the pieces (see appendix). You should be aware that there are a number of free websites where you can learn to make larger pieces on your own (one good suggestion is making the puzzle from foam sections, creating a 3-D puzzle). There are also a number of websites where you can try this activity online. The rules of tangrams are very simple: pieces must be placed flat, you must use all seven pieces, pieces must not overlap, and all pieces must touch each other (though these traditional rules are not always followed). All seven pieces can form several basic shapes (see below). These shapes are a good place to start. I have also provided some additional shapes in the appendix with the hope that you see this activity as fun and recognize the numerous pictures one can make.

Activity One Instructions: Review the rules of tangrams as outlined above before you begin. Now organize the seven pieces in the same order each time before you start. Start a timer or stopwatch and try to complete shape number one as quickly as possible. Record your time. Now move on to shape number two. I would go through these twice in a row so you get a good feel for them. Continue to work on these basic shapes until you see good improvement in your time, then *change* to four other basic shapes or add some picture puzzles. Once you see good improvements in your next set, *change them once again.*

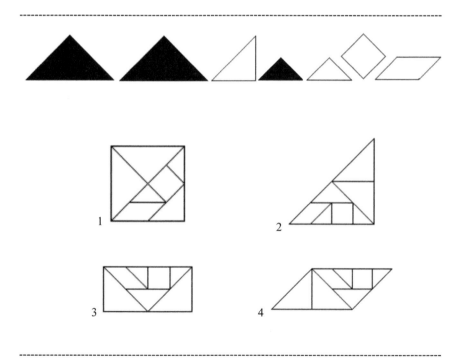

Figure 3.1. *Tangram Puzzle.* (WJ Tippett/*Building an Ageless Mind.* Rowman & Littlefield Publishers, Inc.)

Activity Two—3-D Puzzles

There are a couple of options for this task. I will suggest three ways to perform it, but there are of course a number of ways you can do this type of activity. My suggestion is to purchase either a set of building blocks with the ability to make a number of different simple designs or objects (must come with instructions) or a couple of different simple wooden 3-D puzzle kits (e.g., of animals) from a local craft store. These can also be painted or decorated as well. The third option is to purchase 3-D puzzle kits, which are made of foam and require you to construct famous structures from around the world (e.g., the Eiffel Tower or the CN Tower).

Activity Two Instructions: If you purchase the smaller wooden puzzles, I would use these in a timed task. For example, if these are animals, use three animals each day and time how long it takes to put them together. If you get a basic set of building blocks, use the instructions for making an object and time how quickly you assemble it. Two or three designs should be sufficient. Check your progress at the end of the week. If you are improving, *change* the object you are assembling. For the third option, the 3-D structures can be more of an ongoing activity. With these types of puzzles I would simply set aside a certain amount of time each day (e.g., fifteen to twenty minutes) to work on the puzzle.

Activity Three—Navigation Task

This activity is a great excuse for you to get out and do some shopping or discover a local trail. If your mobility is limited, or you just need a break, there are a couple of alternatives to this task that I will outline below, such as counting shapes or maze finding. I have provided two examples below. Note that you can find puzzles like these online for free or at your local bookstore. These are good alternatives to the navigation task.

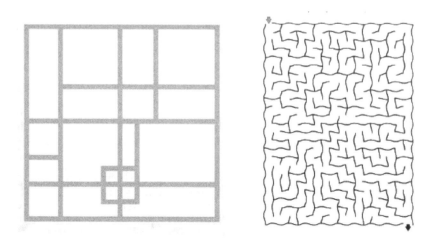

Figure 3.2. *Navigation Task.* (**WJ** Tippett/*Building an Ageless Mind.* **Rowman & Littlefield Publishers, Inc.)**

Alternative Activity Instructions: For the first image, organize squares into three sizes, small, medium, and large. Then provide a total count for all squares and a subtotal for the three sizes. The second image is a basic maze-finding task. You start at one end and work your way to the exit. I suggest timing yourself and recording the number of wrong turns you make. You can rotate a set of twenty mazes (photocopy them), and make sure to organize them so you know how you performed each time you did each maze. Also, rotating through them will ensure the task is varied and challenging.

Activity Three Instructions: If possible, find a local mall, university, art gallery (indoor structures are great in the winter), outdoor trail with lots of twists and turns and different paths, or someplace similar. Go with a friend, family member, or significant other. Ask for a map of the place you are, and then have your friend pick a point on the map and time how long it takes you to get there (also mark how many wrong turns you make so you can compare the next time you try this location). Each week change the spot on the map, but have your partner keep track of the places you have been. After trying five different places, start at the first one again and compare your performance to the last time. You and your friend could also alternate and test each other, which can provide some healthy competition.

4

REASONS NOT TO FORGET THE TEMPORAL LOBE AND HOW WE SEE THE OCCIPITAL LOBE

After reading this chapter, you should be able to answer the following questions:

What types of activities are my temporal and occipital lobes responsible for performing?

What common changes in the temporal and occipital lobes occur as one ages?

What is the importance of the hippocampus in forming memories?

Would damage to the temporal lobe affect my language ability?

As has been shown, the frontal and parietal regions of the brain are responsible for taking the lead in completing many very important tasks on a day-to-day basis. However, without the collaboration of the temporal and occipital lobes a lot of the actions performed by these regions would suffer from a lack of meaning and perspective. The temporal lobe is the area within the brain that controls our emotional responses, memory of events, names of things in our world, sensory systems such as our hearing and seeing, language ability, sexual behavior, and, most importantly for aging individuals, the sense of who we are, our personalities, and responses to events based on our learned experiences. These are just a few of the very important tasks linked to the temporal lobe, but as one can see, it plays an essential role in our ability to function and interact with the world around us in a personally meaningful way. The occipital lobe, though, is not an area rich in meaning; it is one of the basic brain areas that are required to function effectively to support our ability to see and transfer this information to additional brain regions for action. This chapter highlights some of the important functions of the temporal and occipital lobes and examines how and what changes can be observed as an individual ages and how certain subregions respond in the face of a focused deficit.

WHAT ARE THE PRIMARY RESPONSIBILITIES OF THE TEMPORAL LOBE?

To list all of the functions the temporal lobe has been found to perform would take several books. Therefore, in the interest of your time and my space, I will highlight just some important functions of the temporal lobe and how they help us interact with our world. Some of the primary features of the temporal lobe (see figure 2.1) are processing auditory information (via the primary auditory cortex) and aiding in the production of language (i.e., in the Wernicke's and Broca's areas; see figure 4.1). Also, the temporal lobe contains a region called the hippocampus (see figure 4.2), which is primarily implicated in our ability to form, store, and use our memories. Thus, as you can see, this region performs some very important functions.

As we age, the interruption of temporal lobe functions can become quite noticeable (e.g., language or memory issues), which is why testing this area can be very informative to health-care professionals. Why and how these regions are altered as we age will be discussed shortly; however, before I discuss them, I would like to outline how and what specific regions within the temporal lobe contribute to our language and memory processes.

Hearing, speech, and particularly the use of language are the cornerstone of what makes us different from other animals in our world. The temporal lobe contains regions linked to both the production and understanding of language. For example, Broca's area on the left side of the brain in the temporal lobe is known to be responsible for speech production. Thus, when damage occurs to this area, individuals have problems speaking fluently. Individuals with halting and broken speech production could have an illness called Broca's aphasia. Individuals with

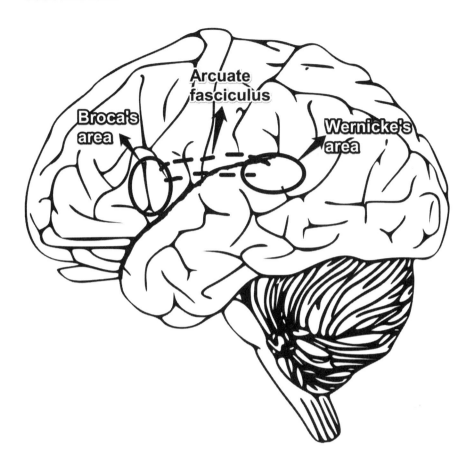

Figure 4.1. *Wernicke's and Broca's Areas.* **(WJ Tippett/***Building an Ageless Mind.***
Rowman & Littlefield Publishers, Inc.)**

Broca's aphasia will retain the ability to understand speech, but producing it becomes quite difficult. On the other hand, individuals with Wernicke's aphasia have no issue with the production of speech, but the
comprehension of it or the producing of proper sentence structure is
primarily affected.[1] Individuals with Wernicke's aphasia also show difficulty in writing with appropriate form and content. Thus, such tasks as
writing a letter can be quite problematic for them. I have highlighted
these communication issues because they are often used as signs that
the brain is experiencing or has undergone an assault in certain areas of
the temporal lobe.

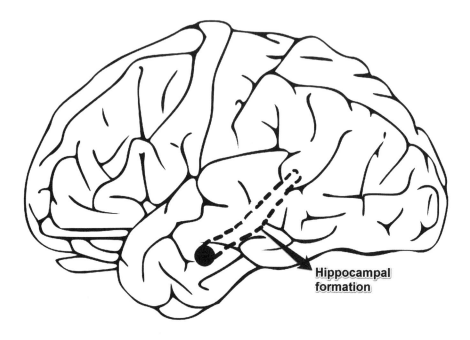

Figure 4.2. *The Hippocampus.* (WJ Tippett/*Building an Ageless Mind.* **Rowman & Littlefield Publishers, Inc.)**

The term *aphasia* is a general term used by health-care professionals to describe those who are experiencing some form of language impairment, be it speaking or written, and generally is accompanied by a disease or injury. Aphasia in general can occur for a number of reasons; one of the most common causes of the onset of aphasia is a stroke episode. In fact, it has been reported that 18 to 38 percent of individuals experiencing a stroke will show symptoms of aphasia.[2] In addition, one of the cognitive features examined in neurodegenerative disease, particularly in the diagnosis of Alzheimer's disease, is the presence of a progressive aphasia deficit.[3] Researchers have shown that the presence of aphasia is very common in individuals with Alzheimer's disease and that the more severe the case of Alzheimer's disease, the more profound the aphasia-type disorder.[4] In fact, it has been shown that to a certain extent most Alzheimer's patients will experience a form of aphasia, with the most likely symptoms related to one's ability to find appropriate words when speaking, name objects, and write properly. As well, many caregivers report these symptoms very early on in the course of the illness.[5] Given these facts, if you have undergone or will undergo cognitive (neuropsychological) testing, you can be assured that your ability to use language will be evaluated. Language impairment, be it word-finding problems, comprehension difficulty, or syntax issues, indicates to clinicians an issue in the left temporal lobe. As noted above, illness related to a neurodegenerative condition such as Alzheimer's disease or having a stroke are highly related to the presence of aphasia.

Interestingly, a key risk factor in the development of Alzheimer's disease and in the chance of one experiencing a stroke-related episode rises with one's age. Thus, as one ages, one can expect the likelihood of experiencing either of these illnesses to increase, consequently increasing the chance of aphasia.

The facts presented above and throughout are not the rule but are simply a description of what is or could be possible as a result of brain trauma. What is also possible is intact and healthy functioning of one's ability driven by the temporal lobe. Just because we age does not mean that we necessarily lose performance ability, and if we work at it, we can maintain our abilities. Strategies for doing so are described throughout this book.

Besides language ability, the temporal lobe performs a number of very important functions. One of the most studied of these functions is one's ability to remember (e.g., faces and places). Memories are a rich source of information for individuals, to the extent that it would be very difficult to operate each and every day without them. Memories are also essential to our sense of who we are. The primary region of focus in regard to our memory is the hippocampus. This brain region has sparked numerous investigations into why our ability to remember becomes impaired, and in some cases why it may be quite excellent and above average.

THE HIPPOCAMPUS

The hippocampus (Greek for "sea horse"; see figure 4.2) is a very important substructure in our temporal lobe and is the primary region where we process and encode information to assist our long-term memory. This is the current standard definition that one can glean from many psychology and health textbooks. However, it is important to note that the hippocampus can also be thought of as a region that helps facilitate the process of remembering by assisting in the storing and retrieval of memories throughout the cerebral cortex. The hippocampus, and more specifically the hippocampal formation and areas closely linked to it, such as the CA1 and the entorhinal cortex, is greatly affected in Alzheimer's disease. This collection of substructures is involved in a process known as "long-term potentiation," whereby axons fire and assist in the formation of memories. This process can also be carried out in other areas of the brain, but to date much of this process is believed to occur in the hippocampus.[6] Research has shown that the hippocampus maintains memories for a limited duration of time, after which many of these are transferred to other brain regions. The ones that are transferred successfully will often be maintained for your lifetime. Identification of the processes the hippocampus performs has also been supported by patient research. For example, one of the most famous cases examining the role and type of processing the hippocampus performs involved an individual named Henry Molaison (aka HM). Henry had the majority of his hippocampus removed in an operation at the age of twenty-seven (in 1953) to help calm his seizures. However, what was not known at the time was how important the hippocampus was in storing and retrieving memories. After the surgery, Henry did not experience any intellectual deficits, but his ability to form new memories was dramatically affected. In fact, Henry often could hold new information for only a short time before it was gone, especially if he got distracted. Henry was always wondering what happened just a few minutes before he got to "his now." Henry was able to maintain some memories from before his surgery, such as how to get home to his old house, but new memories could not be formed.[7] This made Henry the main subject in many studies, and the perfect subject because he never remembered taking part in them. In addition to his amnesia for new events, he lost memories back to about the age of sixteen, causing retrograde amnesia.[8]

Thus, in certain cases of neurodegeneration (e.g., Alzheimer's disease) we assume significant damage to the hippocampal region has occurred based on the disruption observed in memory. These theories are often supported by postmortem examination, during which a brain autopsy shows damage to the hippocampal area. This early realization of the importance of the hippocampus resulted in much research being conducted to date, and the cascading process of memory-related deficits starting from the hippocampal region has also received much attention.

One of the cool things about the hippocampus is that it contains neurons that have been described as "place cells." In one very interesting study, researchers measured the brain activity of people while they walked around a virtual environment. This brain activity was then analyzed via a computer program, and based on the individuals' brain responses (as they walked around) researchers were able to determine where the individuals had been in this virtual environment.[9] Thus, simply by measuring brain activity, they could chart the path of the individual around the virtual room. This type of interface between one's brain and computer is a remarkable advancement in our ability to understand how specific structures can be mapped, and in this case, the extent to which we could determine where an individual has been. This of course raises the questions of where this research can go, and I think the possibilities are quite exciting. For example, what else might we be able to mimic or map as the brain responds to a certain type of activity? Perhaps if we could map our thought process as we worked on a problem or set of problems, this tracking might be important to other intellectual challenges down the road. Thus, if you can imagine, we could have some of the most brilliant researchers wired up every day as they work, in the event that something they thought of that day might be very important to solving future problems. In fact, computer programs could be utilized to demonstrate common bonds between researchers.

WHAT IS THE PRIMARY RESPONSIBILITY OF THE OCCIPITAL LOBE?

The occipital lobe is host to one's primary visual cortex and is responsible for our ability to see. It is divided into two general regions called the striate cortex and extrastriate cortex. The occipital lobe is located at the back of our brain (see figure 2.1) and is responsible for processing the majority of what we see in our world. Visual information is received through our eyes and is transferred to the occipital lobe via the optic nerve. Visual information can also be processed simultaneously in other regions specialized for detecting changes in our visual world; however, to remain on topic I will focus specifically on what goes on within the occipital lobe. The striate cortex is responsible for our ability to process visual information related to movement, form, spatial frequency (intensity of brightness), retinal disparity (different points of view from each eye), and color.[10] Thus, all information is processed on a basic level here, and then as required, it is transferred to the extrastriate cortex or out to other brain regions for help in applying meaning or understanding. The striate cortex sends out signals to additional brain regions and also can receive signals in order to modify what one is observing and help make sense of our world.

An interesting observation is that atrophy within the occipital lobe is linked to the manifestation of visual hallucinations. In fact, researchers have reported that individuals that have a disease such as Alzheimer's are noted to have an increased number of structural abnormalities in the visual association cortex, and consequently the primary type of hallucinations these individuals experience are vision based.[11] As well, specific atrophy within the occipital lobe as a result of vascular issues has been linked to visual hallucinations.[12] Note that atrophy within this region and others is not a normal part of aging, and individuals that experience these types of symptoms should seek medical assistance to determine how and why hallucinations have started. I have provided this as an example of what atrophy in this area could produce; however, the symptoms I have described could also arise for any number of other reasons, and one should be examined before becoming concerned that brain atrophy is automatically present.

IMAGING RESEARCH AND THE TEMPORAL LOBE

The temporal lobe has a very rich history of scientific evaluation, with the modern analysis of this region dating back to the time of Hermann Ebbinghaus and his memory experiments in the late 1800s and early 1900s. More recently, with the advent of our ability to image the brain, greater examination of this region has been undertaken. Because the hippocampus has been the subject of much memory research prior to the development of brain imaging tools, when this technology became more widely available researchers of course wanted to examine the relationship between memory performance and the hippocampus.

What has been shown thus far is that the hippocampus is a leading brain region involved in one's ability to store and encode (process) information. Imaging research has shown that individuals trying to remember a list of words, both initially and then twenty-four hours later, showed activation specifically within the hippocampus.[13] Clinical studies examining populations with irregular brain activity, such as schizophrenic patients, have noted that the ability to recall words freely was impaired by irregular brain activation patterns in the left hippocampal area.[14] Conversely, researchers have also shown that by enhancing the available glucose (a neurotransmitter) in the brain, greater activation could be observed within the hippocampus, resulting in an individual's increased ability to remember emotionally arousing pictures versus individuals who were administered a placebo.[15] The temporal lobe also contains regions linked to one's emotional state and emotional memory. Researchers have shown that when individuals remember certain emotional events, the temporal regions show similar activation patterns to when the events were being experienced.[16] Thus, humans are storing more than memories in their temporal regions; they are also storing emotional responses.

As noted earlier, the temporal lobe plays a very important part in our ability to use language. Because this activity is so important, protecting this area during surgical interventions has been the emphasis of some clinical researchers. Using functional imaging tools, researchers have been able to show which brain regions are highly active during speech production, and a majority of activation for language regions was observed in the anterior temporal lobe. With the use of these functional maps, researchers are able to help guide surgeons when removing brain tissue. This guided surgery significantly reduces the impact on a patient's language and is used to spare essential areas noted to be used in speech production and comprehension. Brain mapping is used frequently in surgeries that require removing brain tissue to help alleviate seizure activity.[17] This type of guided surgery is not unlike the procedure used by Dr. Wilder Penfield at the Montréal Neurological Institute in the mid-twentieth century. Instead of precise imaging-guided procedures, Dr. Penfield would probe the brain to find the area of seizure activity to be removed and map the essential regions around the area to avoid unnecessary damage. Though this was certainly not as precise as these days, the procedure was pioneering work.

In addition to these imaging studies, several other activities have also been noted in the temporal lobe. For example, the temporal lobe has been linked to one's ability to process pictures, sounds, and spoken words and is the primary region involved in neurogenesis (which I will talk about much later).[18]

IMAGING RESEARCH AND THE OCCIPITAL LOBE

Any imaging experiment using the presentation of visual stimuli to study activation in the brain during the performance of a particular task will show activity within the occipital lobe. As well, the occipital lobe is known to be responsible for transferring information back onto several different areas of the brain in order to understand what one is viewing. Thus, it is important to note that imaging research shows that we use the primary visual areas in seeing something, but that we will also send information on to higher cortical regions to help us make sense of what we are seeing. Therefore, there are thousands of research projects using imaging tools that have activated the occipital lobe, confirming that this area is indeed needed to see and make sense of visual items in our world.

Interesting cases arise when an individual has a lesion within the primary visual cortex. If you ask such a person to tell you what he or she can see, the most likely answer will be nothing. However, individuals with this type of damage have shown some ability to detect movement. Though for all intents and purposes they are blind, the fact that they see motion indicates the use of higher visual areas that maintain the ability, on some level, to get visual information from other structures.[19] While the occipital lobe is defined as the primary area for the reception of visual information, it is important to note that due to advances in imaging we know that vision dominates the majority of our cortex in the performance of many tasks. In fact, research on monkey brains has noted that 55 percent of the cortex is dedicated to processing visual information. Thus, visual information from the occipital lobe transfers information to multiple visual regions within the temporal, parietal, and frontal lobes.[20] The integration of this information by these regions is essential for interacting with our external world, and deficits in transferring or integrating this information can prove very detrimental.

BRAIN CHANGES AS WE AGE

In general, excluding a number of abnormal factors affecting brain changes, including overt damage or damage not previously detected such as atrophy related to a specific illness or perhaps a previous stroke, results from research for the most part reflect what one can expect from aging normally. Thus, studies of how the brain changes as one ages remove individuals with significant concerns that might affect the results. Therefore, I will present information related to healthy individuals, and we can therefore assume that this information is not for individuals who have had a significant brain deficit.

Temporal Lobe

First off, in general, individuals fifty and older (age range fifty to eighty-seven) show a significant reduction in their temporal lobe brain matter, a factor directly related to the aging process. Specifically, men, more so than women, display reduction in the middle areas of the temporal lobe as a result of age.[21] Reduction is not restricted to the temporal lobe, but for researchers trying to discount normal aging processes, this region is essential. Why this difference in regard to sex? One theory is that hormones play a factor; specifically, declining testosterone levels might influence this process and have been previously linked to brain weights in the hippocampus in animal experiments. Additionally, when testosterone is administered to aging men, improvements in spatial cognition can be seen. This theory, however, is at best speculative, and much research needs to be conducted to disentangle the effects of a specific hormone versus various environmental factors.[22] Additional research has indicated that it is easy to view male brain reduction as a function of age because of the stable hormone processes that exist for men, as opposed to women, who experience significant changes in their later years. With the onset of menopause, hormone changes abound, and these changes can affect women in their latter years, resulting in a more rapid decline in brain volume than their male counterparts, who experience a stable trajectory.[23]

Thus, it's clear that changes as a result of age can significantly alter our brain processes both structurally and chemically, particularly in the temporal lobe. Though age-related reductions in brain volume of the temporal lobe can be seen, other research suggests this decline increases significantly after the age of seventy.[24] Reductions, however, are tempered by how much of one's brain remains intact and functioning effectively. For instance, on average, men begin with a greater brain volume than women; thus, though reductions are greater for men, especially in the temporal lobe, the remaining temporal lobe structure overall for men still remains larger than women's.[25] How this plays into our ability to process and handle information will be discussed throughout this book. Needless to say, bigger does not necessarily equal better.

Occipital Lobe

The occipital lobe, and specifically the primary visual cortex, does not generally receive much attention when researchers examine brain changes as a result of age. This is because the primary visual cortex is focused primarily on perceiving our world (just seeing, which is actually a highly complex act). Much of the "interesting" functions or dysfunctions related to one's vision are located in higher visual association areas. Damage within the primary visual cortex will simply turn off one's vision. Weakened visual ability as a result of age is normally a physiological issue that occurs outside the brain.

However, researchers interested in overall brain changes include the occipital lobe when trying to determine regional atrophy concerns or in cases of a neurodegenerative condition such as Alzheimer's disease. Researchers generally report that when measuring individuals across age groups at different points in time (e.g., at forty, sixty, and seventy) or following individuals over a period of time (e.g., five years), results indicated little to no change in the size of the occipital lobe.[26] Therefore, as we age, we can expect to "see" little difference in our occipital lobe and little effect on our vision as a result of alterations within our brain.

TRAINING THE TEMPORAL LOBE

As mentioned earlier, the temporal lobe contains a number of highly specific subregions involved in some of our most complex abilities. It has areas involved in our ability to organize sensory information, including our ability to speak and hear. It also contains areas tied to our ability to process and assist in storing information for later recall. It is noted to contain areas directly related to our general memory abilities. And it contains regions involved with our ability to perceive and provide meaning to objects in our world. In addition to these abilities, the temporal lobe is linked to our emotional processing. In short, the temporal lobe is the region of the brain that makes us, us.

Damage or disruptions within the temporal lobe can cause problems in one's ability to speak and comprehend speech; the ability to remember events, names, faces, and objects; the processing of emotions; learning; attention; and many other functions. Though much of this region spontaneously performs these functions for us, such as our ability to understand speech and respond appropriately, some other areas require more hands-on involvement. One of these hands-on tasks is the ability to remember, though we should not forget that we store a significant amount of information without any effort, such as how we find our way home each day or the names of our parents or siblings.

However, as we age, we must learn new things and ways to successfully interact with the world around us. For example, attending school requires us daily to remember various amounts of information that may not possess much internal meaning. This type of activity can be quite difficult, and trying to retain this type of information can require significant effort for some individuals. This effort challenges the brain. However, after we finish formal education and secure employment, many of the tasks we learn can become routine, and we start to know the answer to every question related to our occupation as we confront the same issues over and over again. Many individuals relish this opportunity and often enjoy not having to learn so much extraneous information on a daily basis. Others might choose a career path that requires significant learning of new activities, information, procedures, and the like, and thus they are unknowingly helping to keep their brain fit. If in the past few weeks you were required to learn a new set of procedures, a new language, or some information that you wanted to share with others, you were engaging in activities that were undoubtedly stimulating your temporal lobe. It is important to note that using working memory for activities like remembering a phone number until you dial it, though it certainly involves the temporal lobe, does not have a significant ongoing consequence for this region. Thus, in an effort to ensure that individuals are engaging in activities that are directly related to the temporal lobe, and to ensure the ongoing engagement of this region, I have provided some activities to help "exercise" and activate this area. Below are some activities individuals can use to target the temporal lobe. The overall goal in all of these activities is to ensure individuals have choices and an understanding of the different types of tasks one should take part in to prevent or rehabilitate cognitive concerns related to this region.

TEMPORAL LOBE ACTIVITIES

The tasks below will ensure the activation of the temporal lobe. Though all of these activities activate similar areas, the pathways used to complete such tasks have been shown to be quite different.[27] Thus, these activities provide the best of both worlds, in that they activate major temporal regions as well as additional pathways within and outside of the temporal lobe. Multiple imaging studies show that learning or recalling words, as well as remembering stories or events for later retrieval, such as in the storytelling involved in activity two, is linked directly to temporal subregions.[28] As for the final activity, it has been shown that producing, processing, or learning a language activates many regions of the temporal lobe and, as such, is an excellent temporal lobe activity.[29]

Activity One—Memory Training

This first task comes from the German psychologist Hermann Ebbinghaus, who was one the first researchers to examine human memory. One of his very early experiments involved his creating thousands of three-letter nonsense words consisting of a consonant, a vowel, and a consonant. Ebbinghaus would make a list of a few, then read them out loud and attempt to remember them in the order he read them. He would write them down and each day try to remember the order correctly and check himself over the passing days to see how well he did.

Activity One Instructions: Take a piece of paper and make a row of three-letter nonsense words that include a consonant, a vowel, and a consonant (e.g., BOK, KIB, JOR). After you make this list, check it over to ensure the words are nonsense words and do not represent something meaningful. You could start with a list of ten nonsense words. Read the words out loud and work to remember them. You can do this in the morning and then put the list away, and then in the afternoon see how many you can remember. Again, depending on your ability, you can change both how many words to remember and also how much time to give yourself between learning the list and recalling the words.

Activity Two—Storytelling

One of our great abilities as experiential learners is being able to recount events that have occurred, particularly those that have provided us with meaning or a moral. Ensuring that events follow an appropriate sequence is essential in these types of tales and, thus, use significant resources within the temporal lobe.

Activity Two Instructions: There are two ways to approach this activity, and I would suggest trying both. The first is to write down a story that you have learned a lesson from. Make sure it is not too long, and include important details such as colors, names, and places that you can use as markers to check how much you remember accurately. Write down these important marker points and add them up. You can use this as a score to see how well you are doing. Once you have constructed this story, retell it to yourself or to a friend and have them check the details as you go. If needed, you can ask for some prompts and see how many marker points you cover (deduct half a point for using a prompt). Try this until you get good at telling the story, and then *change it*. Write another one and start over again.

The second option is to find a short story with a moral and meaning and enough detail to create marker points. Learn the story and then try retelling it, describing it in as much detail as possible while ensuring you cover each marker point (which you will have identified ahead of time). This second option might help get you started if you have difficulty creating one of your own. Once you get good at retelling this story, *change it up* and find a new one.

Activity Three—Foreign Language

When individuals learn a language, their brains work to create associations (with, for example, names of objects, actions, etc.). Many of us learn our language at a very young age and create many of these associations during a period of significant brain development (neurogenesis). Though much of the brain is at work during this period, the temporal lobe plays a very important role in creating these associations and in reproducing and comprehending the language. If you are concerned that I am about to suggest that you learn a new language, don't worry. I do not think you need to go to that extent. It would be very beneficial if you gave it a try, but if you are concerned about your ability here is a scaled-down version.

Activity Three Instructions: Pick a foreign language that you have an interest in. Picking a language that is of interest to you will help you maintain focus on this task. Create pictures for items you wish to learn the words to in that language. Keep the words on the pictures for a while and in places around the house where you will see them often. Work on pronouncing the words and practice rehearsing how to say them for each item. Keep these posted until you feel you have a handle on the words, and then remove them and over the next few days name the pictures using the foreign-language words. Once again, after you have learned these names, start with a new set of pictures and words.

Summary

Though I have proposed several activities in this and previous chapters to activate distinct brain areas, I need to add one note of caution. Flexibility and novelty are reasons the brain works harder and are shown to increase overall activation. If a task becomes routine, the brain will not need as many resources to perform it. Therefore, you need to continually change the types of activities you engage in. If you become very proficient at one type of activity, then change it. Individuals will often state that they do their crossword every day, "so my brain gets exercise." I often ask if they are good at it, and the answer is normally yes. But they are good at it because it has become routine and does not require as many resources as doing a crossword for the very first time. Thus, individuals need to be aware that novel tasks are very important for brain health. The above tasks are provided as a guide to how one can activate certain brain regions. These tasks are only suggestive, and I am certain there are many other tasks that could be beneficial. The point is to ensure you are engaging in a variety of tasks, and if you want to change the type of task, make sure you do research to understand which areas of the brain will be involved. Overall brain health will require overall brain involvement.

5

WHAT IS COGNITIVE RESERVE AND HOW IMPORTANT IS IT IN MAINTAINING A HEALTHY BRAIN?

After reading this chapter, you should be able to answer the following questions:

What is a cognitive reserve?
How does my lifestyle affect my cognitive ability?
What is the role of education in protecting my brain as I age?
What are the effects of having a challenging career on my brain health?
What is neurogenesis?

COGNITIVE RESERVE

Cognitive reserve is a broadly used term that refers to one's general ability to create a strong, healthy brain that can handle adverse events. Cognitive reserve is often observed in individuals who have a high IQ, a challenging occupation, a high level of education, and a history of participation in challenging leisure activities. These processes are thought to lead to better "neural processing" (e.g., more efficient brain use and better brain capacity) and help build a cognitive reserve that may not be present in individuals without these attributes. As noted, individuals with cognitive reserve often demonstrate a greater ability to handle adverse brain pathology (e.g., disease states such as Alzheimer's disease [AD]) and can use this reserve ability to compensate for structural deficits to complete desired behavioral and functional responses. If you are reading this and you have a high school diploma or less, or do not have a very challenging job, you might feel that you are doomed, but do not fear—you're not! In fact, taking an interest in changing your current brain state for the better at any stage will be beneficial to you. For example, I believe that just reading this book and working with the strategies outlined in many of the chapters is a great way to help boost your cognitive reserve. Besides the activities in the other chapters, I have also outlined some tips for you at the conclusion of this chapter. In order to convince you that having or building a cognitive reserve is very important, I've provided some evidence to inspire you to get going, or to maintain ability if you have already built a good foundation.

The cognitive reserve hypothesis suggests that having a high cognitive reserve leads to a more "flexible" or "malleable" brain that can handle changes related to neuropathology (biological diseases such as AD) or vascular damage (changes in brain structure and blood vessel structure), which often delays many individuals from displaying, noticing, and reporting any significant cognitive impairments. In fact, many "high cognitive" individuals may die without even experiencing any significant disruptions in their cognitive performance (even though, anatomically, their brains might be adversely affected), which would be ideal for the majority of us.

THE EDUCATION FACTOR

One of the primary questions researchers often examine is if increased education can protect cognition (thought processes) as one ages. The principal way this question can be examined is through epidemiological (population) research. Epidemiological research is one of our best sources of information as it relates to tracking levels of education, death rates, cognitive impairments, age, and so on. One recent study in the United States examined education levels as determinates of cognitive impairment in individuals age fifty-five and older. This research showed that educated men and women benefit greatly from their higher levels of education, as measured through reduced rates of cognitive impairment as they aged. Higher education in this study referred to those with a college degree, and lower education individuals were those with less than a high school education. Results from this study demonstrated that white women and men had a 10 percent increased lifetime rate of experiencing a cognitive impairment if they were in the lower education group. Black men and women were shown to have the greatest chance of experiencing a cognitive impairment if they were in the low education group, with lifetime rates of 49 percent for the women and 57 percent for the men. These values suggest that education is playing a significant role in reducing symptoms related to cognitive impairment. Though the goal is to always control for socioeconomic factors, we should keep in mind that the results could be influenced based on an individual's life status. As well, these authors identified that higher education was linked to increases in life expectancy. The study noted that highly educated men lived 1.6 fewer years with a cognitive impairment than those in the low education group. Highly educated women were reported to live 1.9 fewer years without cognitive impairment than women with less education.[1]

Interestingly, these researchers also examined factors like smoking and body mass index (BMI) related to cognitive impairment and life expectancy. Not surprisingly, factors that increased lifespan included being a woman and not smoking. However, the ultimate point was that only individuals with higher levels of education were shown to have a reduced rate of cognitive impairment as they advanced in age. Though BMI was not shown to play a role in cognition, smoking did in one respect. These researchers explained that if you are a smoker, the good news is you will experience less time with a cognitive impairment; the bad news is you are expected to die much sooner (hence the less time with a cognitive impairment). To summarize, this research clearly links education and cognitive decline, but it does not disentangle education levels from individuals with good cognitive habits or those with cognitively challenging careers.

HIGH COGNITIVE LIFESTYLE

A UK study has suggested that individuals aged sixty-five to eighty-one with a "high cognitive lifestyle" score, computed by looking at education and level of engagement with complex mental activities, had a decreased risk of moving from no to slight impairment. These individuals also had a greater ability to bounce back to a nonimpaired state after a period of impairment. This study also showed that if those with a high cognitive lifestyle were in a severely impaired state, they had a greater risk of mortality.[2] I believe this point shows that people with a high cognitive lifestyle can combat impairment so effectively and for such a long time that when they reach a severe state of impairment, they have unknowingly already experienced a significant amount of damage to their brain, which may result in their reaching a tipping point where they can no longer ease the effects of a "brain attack," resulting in the full force of the attack being brought to bear on the individual. The primary finding of the UK study was that if you engage in a high cognitive lifestyle, you are more likely to have better cognitive health as you age and a greater ability to respond to cognitive challenges.[3]

Additional research examining diseases and trauma in aging individuals suggests that effects can be reduced as a result of one's level of education or occupational attainment. In fact, one study has shown this through an examination of 249 participants with identified "brain burden" as a result of either a cerebrovascular incident (i.e., stroke) or an Alzheimer's disease–type pathology.[4] Individuals were less likely to experience symptoms related to their illness if they had attained a greater level of education or had a higher "grade" of occupation. It is important to note that these researchers used population census data and did not make fine distinctions as to what is deemed a cognitively challenging occupation. Instead, they used classification factors such as "managerial or professional" to determine high-grade occupations, which is a very broad classification system. One can certainly have a professional occupation but still engage in the same routine each and every day. Thus, though the occupation may be deemed "professional," the activities of that occupation can become mundane and unchallenging. I would like to provide an example at this point. However, out of fear of receiving thousands of letters explaining to me how a certain job is very challenging, I will leave it to you to determine and discuss with your friends.

BRAIN STRUCTURE, BILINGUALISM, AND COGNITIVE RESERVE

Research examining brain structure and cognitive reserve has suggested that individuals with a greater cognitive reserve have, in general, larger brains and reduced brain activity when performing tasks. Though "reduced brain activity" sounds like a bad thing, it is thought to occur because healthy individuals use their "brain resources" more efficiently. Research on this topic shows that individuals with a higher cognitive reserve who are experiencing mild cognitive impairment or AD demonstrate greater brain volume than those individuals with no reserve.[5] Thus, the actual anatomical brain structure can affect cognitive ability, and individuals with a greater cognitive reserve will fair much better structurally as they age, even if confronted by a disease.

This structural brain advantage (i.e., increased brain areas critical for ensuring an adequate level of functioning) has also been observed in individuals who are fluently bilingual. Research has shown that bilingual individuals with AD have a significant reduction in brain size in regions noted to be associated with AD pathology. Even though this group had greater brain atrophy in critical brain regions, they showed cognitive ability similar to their monolingual counterparts who had less brain atrophy. The authors believe that bilingualism is a factor that can contribute to the delaying of symptoms related to cognitive impairment, and that these bilingual individuals can function at higher-than-expected levels in the face of greater brain atrophy.[6] Additionally, work prior to this examination concluded that the symptoms of AD can be significantly delayed, possibly by as much as five years, in individuals who possess bilingual ability.[7] Thus, it appears that a great way to increase your cognitive reserve and efficient brain functioning is to use a second language as much as possible. This could be viewed as a way to "flex" your brain, keeping it active and healthy.

I would also suggest that learning a new language late in life might help build "network" brain connections. The novelty of learning new words could create a situation where your brain needs to adapt and grow and develop new avenues to be successful. I am not aware of any direct evidence that shows learning a new language late in life will specifically delay cognitive impairment by this many months or this many years, but the alternative would be to do nothing. But as they say, nothing ventured, nothing gained. I believe that activating the brain in many different ways, which could include acquiring a new language, is undoubtedly beneficial in most cases and, as we have seen above, may in fact positively alter cognitive performance.

COGNITIVE RESERVE AND IQ

Does having a higher IQ affect cognitive impairment as one ages? Thus far, the suggestion is that education appears to be the path to ensuring better cognitive vitality as one ages. However, there has been research showing that IQ can have an effect on cognitive performance. The main issue in examining the influence of IQ is trying to untangle it from a person's achieved level of education and careers. As you can imagine, if you have a higher-than-average IQ, you will gravitate toward a more challenging career path, and having a strong desire to learn can result in higher educational attainment.

One study examined the presence of dementia and mild cognitive impairment in relation to an individual's level of IQ as measured in adolescence. The authors controlled for education and sex (thus these variables were removed from influencing the outcome). What they found was that persons with a high IQ in adolescence showed a lower risk of developing dementia or mild cognitive impairment (MCI) as they aged. In addition, the authors pointed out that the greater the activity level (gathered from yearbook data) individuals had in their youth, the fewer incidents of dementia or MCI they reported later in life.[8] This study, of course, has a number of limitations, such as no way to account for the activity level of individuals outside of school activities. As well, using a telephone survey to diagnose the presence of dementia (as was used in this study) is not a sound way to determine such a level of cognitive impairment. Nevertheless, the findings are very interesting and suggest that having a high IQ can be beneficial as one ages. I would offer one further thought on this research: individuals with a higher-than-average IQ are interested in a number of varying topics and cognitive activities, and as such it might be the ongoing engagement in these activities that helps them maintain a healthy brain. In addition, the study noted that individuals who participated in several activities in school also showed better protection from cognitive impairment as they aged. Again, it may not be the early engagement in these activities but rather a natural personality trait that most likely continues throughout adulthood, when engaging in new and varied activities keeps the brain engaged and challenged. If, in fact, it is this ongoing engagement, as I suggest, influencing a healthy cognitive state, then the good news is that it would never be too late to begin.

CAN A CHALLENGING CAREER FILL THE GAP?

One very important question individuals often ask is this: is a formal education a must to ensure good cognitive health, or could a challenging career fill the gap?

In part, to answer this question, I would like to highlight some research from a study on London taxi drivers. Taxi drivers as a study group typically offer good representation of the general public. Sixteen participated in this research, with an average age of forty-four and the oldest participant being sixty-two. Using a control group (people who are not taxi drivers), researchers examined the brains of these two populations to see if they could identify any structural differences in brain size.[9] Surprisingly, what they found was greater brain volume in the posterior hippocampus (a region involved with our ability to perform memory tasks associated with navigation). Furthermore, the longer someone was a taxi driver in London, the greater the volume in this brain region. This research indicates that neural plasticity is a very real component of our ability to adapt to life challenges and can be observed through actual changes in brain structure. As well, increased ability in this case was linked directly to brain changes. Thus, one could suggest that the nature of the work, which does not require several years of education or an outstanding IQ, is nevertheless actively involved in creating neural plasticity and neural growth in the brain. This finding is very exciting news for those who, for whatever reason, did not have the opportunity to be formally educated, but who nevertheless have very challenging careers. It could be that these careers are keeping these individuals cognitively sharp. As well, this research highlights the important fact that, with ongoing effort, all individuals have the ability to alter their brain structure and their cognitive abilities, changes that can be long lasting. To what extent this translates to other regions of the brain is difficult to say, but the evidence appears very promising and would suggest that activating all regions would be of the most benefit.

Studies examining occupation and cognitive performance have been undertaken by a number of researchers. One study evaluated 357 individuals, 122 of whom had Alzheimer's disease. Individuals were interviewed about their occupations and occupational traits throughout their work lives (e.g., in their twenties, thirties, forties, and fifties). The researchers found that occupational traits change throughout the course of one's lifetime, and by statistically controlling for these changes, they believed they could show that occupational traits and occupations that require higher mental ability throughout one's work life are related to a reduced chance of experiencing AD. The results of the research did in fact support this theory, and these researchers were able to show that the more mentally challenging the occupation and the occupational traits, the smaller the chance of being afflicted with a cognitive impairment. Occupations that required high physical demands but had low mental challenge created situations where individuals had a greater susceptibility to cognitive impairment as they aged.[10] These conclusions were in line with other studies and help support the suggestion that those with manual occupations are at a greater risk for dementia-related disturbances.[11] This suggests, then, that occupations that are mentally demanding offer a greater benefit to ensuring cognitive health as we age. However, what is missing is some insight into what these individuals are doing after they are done working. I would contend that individuals that have challenging careers enjoy challenging activities well into their retirement years, and this may be a greater factor for determining how they fair cognitively as they age.

Though now you may be concerned if you have not had a challenging career, and as such have an increased susceptibility to experiencing a cognitive impairment, do not fear! This is certainly not a deciding factor, and it does not mean you will ultimately have a cognitive impairment. There are many individuals who have held manual occupations but still enjoy challenging leisure activities. Interestingly enough, researchers have shown that individuals who engage in certain types of leisure activities are less susceptible to experiencing cognitive impairments as they age. For example, individuals who learn a new skill, study a new subject, and practice mentally challenging problems in their leisure time are known to have a significantly reduced chance cognitive impairment as they age.[12] This evidence is good news for individuals with manual jobs and limited opportunities for a mentally stimulating workday. Spending your leisure time actively engaged in stimulating activities could be of great cognitive benefit as you age. In addition, it highlights the claim I have been making throughout this book that activities need to be novel and ever changing, and that actively seeking out new activities that require a learning phase can be of great cognitive benefit.

Before I move on to tips for creating a good cognitive reserve, I would just like to highlight some scientific evidence about why and how cognitive reserve is created. To do this, I want to briefly discuss the concept of neurogenesis. Neurogenesis is the process whereby our brain produces neurons. This process occurs significantly during the brain's development, but it can also occur in adulthood and is generally limited to certain areas of the brain (e.g., the subgranular zone and the dentate gyrus). However, if one experiences some form of brain trauma, then neurogenesis can occur in these damaged regions. This plasticity is often observed in stroke patients, wherein they begin to regain a significant amount of lost ability in the early days following their stroke event. How does neural plasticity fit with the cognitive reserve phenomenon? One suggestion is that when our brains produce more and more neurons, we create a neurogenic reserve. It is important to note that we all possess the ability for neural growth. Many new neurons die off because we often don't need them unless we are engaged in learning new things. As a result these cells do not accumulate or find an appropriate home. Thus, actively engaging in some form of new learning creates growth and allows new connections to develop. Because we have created a number of new connections, we see actual anatomical growth (like in our London taxi driver example). What this might mean for an individual is that if his or her brain becomes "challenged" (i.e., affected by disease or trauma), he or she has additional resources via additional neural connections to handle these events, creating alternative "routes" or "connections," with the goal of completing a desired behavioral activity and with limited or less stress on our brains.[13]

Now you might be thinking, "This is all well and fine for younger individuals, but I am much older, and I'm sure this does not work in the same way for me." Well, to a certain extent, this is true; it does not work in the same way because as one gets older the process slows. however, the process does not disappear. One's stem cells remain capable of growing and creating new connections throughout one's life.[14] Thus, one might suggest that old dogs can learn new tricks—they just need to work at it a little bit longer.

TIPS FOR CREATING A GOOD COGNITIVE RESERVE

The best way to create a good cognitive reserve is by creating an environment where the process of neurogenesis can flourish. There are a number of ways one can do this. For example, we know that physical exercise can stimulate growth, and an enriched environment can also effect brain change. Thus, having a number of exciting and challenging activities around your house can be beneficial for your brain. Having the opportunity to learn new things is an excellent way to stimulate growth. In addition, just trying new activities in general is a great way to help boost your cognitive reserve. I would also like to highlight that a good cognitive reserve occurs when we develop good habits, so finding a routine that includes novel activities can be an excellent way to ensure you stay on track.

All these suggestions can be very helpful, but it is important to remember that in creating this type of environment you should also strive to limit processes that are bad for your brain. Things such as too much stress can create hormones that are bad for neurogenesis. Not engaging in new activities will limit your ability to create a good cognitive reserve.

One final tip is to find a group or a friend to pick you up at a predetermined time and day to participate in a predetermined activity (e.g., taking a class, or perhaps a new mentally stimulating game or activity). This is a good way to ensure you stay on track and possibly inspire yourself to prepare each week for a new challenge.

Section II

Aging and Disease

6

ALZHEIMER'S DISEASE

After reading this chapter, you should be able to answer the following questions:

What is Alzheimer's disease?
Why do people get Alzheimer's disease?
How is Alzheimer's disease diagnosed?
Does Alzheimer's disease affect my sex life?
Is there a way to prevent Alzheimer's disease?

WHAT IS ALZHEIMER'S DISEASE?

Alzheimer's Disease (AD) is characterized as a neurodegenerative brain disorder of unknown origin, causing progressive memory loss or loss of other mental functions, such as difficulty performing familiar tasks, disorientation to time and place, visuomotor and motor deficits, and word-finding difficulty. Much of these criteria for identifying the illness were developed in 1984 by the National Institute of Neurological and Communicative Disorders and Stroke (NINCDS) and the Alzheimer's Disease and Related Disorders Association (ADRDA).[1] After twenty-seven years, the criteria were updated to reflect the knowledge we have acquired about the disease since. The changes help with diagnosis and in defining variants of the disease, focusing on the impact dementia and AD have on individuals. The main change involved understanding that individuals can present with varying cognitive issues. Some individuals experiencing AD have intact memory ability while displaying other cognitive problems such as a language issue (e.g., word-finding difficulty), visuospatial deficits (e.g., way-finding ability), or deficits in reasoning or problem solving. Memory issues, of course, are still the major concern in many cases, but these other cognitive concerns are now more closely examined. It is also important to note that these deficits must have occurred gradually, without sudden on-set.[2] In the "Diagnosing AD" section of this chapter, I will explain the new categorical breakdown of individuals with AD and discuss the components of each.

On the whole, people affected by AD are interested in what is primarily involved with this disease, but they may also be interested in how common the disease is within a given population. There are varying estimates of what percentage of dementia cases are specifically AD. Alzheimer's Disease International identifies Alzheimer's disease as accounting for 50 to 75 percent of all reported cases of dementia. The high rate often results in individuals believing that dementia and Alzheimer's disease are interchangeable terms, but they are not. In recent years the dementia illness known as vascular dementia has grown in diagnosis and is currently the second most common dementia state. However, I believe within the next few years significant connections to the presence of vascular issues in all dementia patients will be identified, and thus a mixed presentation of the disease will be noted as much more common and diagnosed at a higher rate than AD alone. It is important to keep in mind when hearing the term *dementia* that it is a generic description. An individual could be afflicted with various dementia-related illnesses, such as AD, vascular dementia, Lewy body dementia, frontotemporal dementia, and primary progressive aphasia. The goal, however, of this chapter is to examine AD in detail.

Although a description of AD was given at the beginning of this chapter, the symptoms of the illness can vary significantly from one individual to the next. Historically, memory loss as it relates to day-to-day events has been one of the defining features clinicians look for when trying to determine the presence of dementia. But this is not necessarily the case. The process of diagnosis is, of course, much more involved; the point to be made here is that difficulty with short-term memory, in particular, is very noticeable to family members (probably because of the frustration it causes for them). Family members are on the front lines and are typically aware of when an individual begins to change dramatically. This change is often observed many years after the disease began.

The question many individuals want answered is what specifically is going on in the brain that causes AD.

GENETIC COMPONENTS OF AD

There are two primary genetic processes at work in Alzheimer's disease: the development of neuritic plaques and neurofibrillary tangles.

Neuritic Plaques

Neuritic plaques are generally the result of the accumulation and development of abnormal proteins. These plaques consist of a dense core of proteins known as a beta-amyloid. Beta-amyloid plaques develop because of abnormal cuts to an amyloid precursor protein (APP); this protein is thought to be initially present in neurons for health benefits (e.g., neuron growth). However, the protein is located partially in and outside of the cell. As a result, it gets cut into fragments by enzymes called alpha-, beta-, and gamma-secretase. Plaques are created depending on which protein does the cutting and where the cut occurs on the protein. In the development of AD, the beta-secretase cuts an APP at one end, and gamma-secretase cuts the remaining section at the other end, releasing this section out into the space outside the neuron rather than having it remain within the cell. This is a beneficial and natural path of this process. This beta-amyloid peptide, which has now been released outside of the neuron, is a defective, long-form mutation consisting of forty-two to forty-three amino acids, instead of the intended forty. These long-form beta-amyloid proteins then begin to stick together with other similar proteins. The brain has a process where it can clear some of these abnormal proteins out, but not all of them can or are cleared from the brain, resulting in insoluble "clumps" (or protofibrils). As this process continues, these clumps develop into plaques that are typical of AD.[3] These plaques slow neuron transmission, and the brain sees them as degenerative sections. It then begins a process whereby the cells affected by plaques are enveloped and cleared from the brain. This is a reactive process wherein the brain is doing its best to protect itself. However, the resulting effect is the reduction of neurons and a reduced ability to transmit messages throughout the brain. What remains is a dense set of plaques and a shrinking brain.

Neurofibrillary Tangles

The second major process to be identified in individuals with AD is the development of neurofibrillary tangles. While plaques begin outside of the neuron cell membrane, a neurofibrillary tangle is a process that begins inside the cell. Inside our cells we have a system of microtubules that is like a long string of balloons tied together. This stringlike structure stretches throughout the cell, helping with the transport of cellular nutrients. The protein tau helps bind the microtubules together (like the string from balloon to balloon, keeping them together). What happens in AD is that the molecular structure of tau begins to break down, and as a result a process called hyperphosphorylation occurs. Hyperphosphorylation happens because phosphate ions become attached to the strands of tau. This is bad, because it results in tau losing its ability to bind together microtubules. Thus, the microtubules lose their structure and break apart. This means that the cell does not have a way to feed itself. Eventually, this results in cell death, and what is left in its place is a neurofibrillary tangle.[4]

As you can see, the production of plaques and tangles are very disruptive to the health of one's neuronal structure. Thus, from a genetic perspective, AD is an attack specifically on one's brain cells, from within and from outside of the cell. The result is significant disruptions or complete silence (as a result of cell death) in neural transmission. However, it is important to note that the brain is very resilient, and in many cases there can be significant damage while one's performance remains stable. This happens because our brains find different pathways along which to send and receive messages. How long one can compensate for this ongoing attack varies for a number of reasons that are discussed throughout this book. Researchers have spent many years unravelling the processes I have just described. The goal in understanding what is occurring within an AD brain is to find ways to alter and repair this process. Though to date there is no cure for AD, there have been several advances in modifying these processes, and at the conclusion of this chapter I will report on a few upcoming therapies that hope to alter or stop this process altogether.

WHY DO PEOPLE GET ALZHEIMER'S DISEASE?

This question is very easy to answer: we just do not know, for the most part, how and what causes this process to be triggered. I have qualified this statement by saying "for the most part" because we are unsure of what causes the process to begin in sporadic cases. But in a small number of cases, we know that the disease can be inherited. Thus, AD is often divided into two broad types: hereditary/familial AD and sporadic AD.

The term *sporadic AD* means that there is no identified connection to the cause of the illness. Thus, if one has sporadic AD, it is assumed that there is no hereditary component involved, and the disease has developed without a familial link. Sporadic AD is the most common form and accounts for 80 to 95 percent of AD cases.[5] Suggestions for what causes the sporadic process to be triggered are numerous. For example, there are theories related to head injury, hypertension, heart disease, smoking, diabetes, obesity, cerebrovascular disease, and vitamin deficiencies (e.g., B12, C, E).[6] There is much research in this area, working to determine how and why some individuals get the illness while others do not. However, one of the best determinates of getting AD is simply one's age. As one gets older, the chance of being affected by the illness increases. It has been reported that between the ages of sixty-five and eighty-five one is fifteen times more likely to experience a dementia-related illness.[7]

Genetically, sporadic AD has been linked to a gene on chromosome 19 called the APO E. The APO E gene is encoded for a protein called apolipoprotein E. One of the interesting functions of apolipoprotein E is moving cholesterol in and out of human cells. There are three forms of the APO E gene that have garnered much attention: APO E2, E3, and E4. Every human has two copies of this gene, one from each parent. E3 is reported to be very common, occurring in 40 to 90 percent of the population, whereas E2 is found in 2 percent and E4 in 6 to 37 percent of the population.[8] Interestingly, research has shown that E2 carriers are less likely than the other carrier types to experience AD.

One of the suggestions for why this may be is that E2 gene carries are more likely to have greater cortical thickness. Thus, a thicker cortex can be viewed as a neuroprotective effect against the onset or progression of AD.[9]

As you can see, in regard to sporadic AD, there is currently no definitive evidence to explain why one individual develops AD and another does not. The most well-known fact associated with sporadic AD is that it often has a late onset, meaning that individuals who develop this form of AD often do so after the age of sixty-five. The onset of the familial form of the disease can occur well before the age of sixty-five.

Specific gene mutations have been linked to the familial form (also called early-onset or autosomal-dominant AD), including the genes APP (amyloid precursor protein), PSEN1, and PSEN2 (PSEN stands for *presenilin*).[10] The contribution of each of these genes to the development of AD is complex to say the least. APP, as described earlier, is involved in abnormal cutting of beta-amyloid, which has a higher rate of causing the formation of plaques. Note also that APP is said to account for 10 to 15 percent of familial cases.[11] The mean age of disease onset for individuals with PSEN1 mutation was 41.7 years, showing up in 66 percent of familial cases.[12] The PSEN2 gene mutation is linked to an average age of onset at sixty-two years and has not been reported beyond familial research.[13] The upside of these investigations is that researchers have developed a good understanding of why this group, in particular, has developed AD, unlike individuals with the sporadic form of the illness. It should also be pointed out that individuals who are E4 carriers have a higher rate of the familial form of AD than other forms.[14]

Individuals with familial AD are faced with a very uncomfortable scenario for a couple of reasons. First, they will normally develop AD much earlier than individuals with the sporadic form. Typically, individuals are affected in their forties, fifties, and sixties, though there are reports that it can start even earlier. Second, individuals with early-onset AD progress much faster than those with late-onset AD.[15] For these two reasons alone, one can see that this form of the disease can have a significant effect on one's life. It is important to highlight, though, that even if one has the familial form of AD, it does not guarantee early disease development, despite the increased risk.

DIAGNOSING AD

Diagnosing AD has historically been difficult because showing that an individual was afflicted with neuritic plaques and neurofibrillary tangles could only occur during postmortem examination. In recent years, methods have been developed to determine the presence of these biochemical processes before death (antemortem). Though researchers have had some success in developing these mechanisms,[16] they are still is not entirely definitive. The reason individuals still cannot receive a clear-cut diagnosis of AD until death is that there are many other factors that can result in neuritic plaques and neurofibrillary tangles in the brain.[17] As such, a diagnosis of AD due to dementia comes in one of three ways: probable AD, possible AD, and probable or possible AD (including evidence of a pathophysiological process). This last designation is meant to be used for research purposes.[18] Let's look at what each of these labels imply about one's condition.

Probable AD dementia is diagnosed when individuals first meet "all-cause dementia criteria." These are defined by a number of categories, beginning with identifying if the disease is interfering with the ability to function at work or the completion of one's usual activities. This level of function has to show a noticeable decline and cannot be explained by a psychiatric disorder. A clear history of decline is identified from a credible source and, where possible, via cognitive assessment.

The cognitive and behavioral impairments must include two cognitive domains from the following:

1. Difficulty retaining new information, which is often noticed by caregivers because the individual becomes repetitive in their questions; problems locating regular places; and missing appointments due to memory issues.
2. Problems reasoning or completing multisequence tasks (e.g., making and eating lunch); difficulty planning to perform certain tasks (e.g., a trip to the store) or understanding safety issues while engaging in certain activities; and difficulty managing finances.
3. Problem with visuospatial ability. For example, individuals can exhibit problems using household items (e.g., scissors) and remembering common faces or places.

4. Language concerns, which can include word-finding issues, speaking at a normal pace (e.g., hesitated speech), newfound reading and writing difficulties.
5. Alterations in one's personality or regular behavior. For example, lack of interest in interacting socially, loss of interest in activities, and being noticeably upset.[19]

The preceding information includes the new criteria outlined by McKhann and colleagues and must be met before moving on to the three categories of AD.

Probable AD

Probable AD dementia is diagnosed when the above symptoms are present and the criteria are met. In addition to this, individuals with probable AD will demonstrate the onset of symptoms over time (e.g., a few months or even years). As well, there has to be some record of a significant cognitive decline as observed in either amnestic (memory related concerns) or nonamnestic (memory not affected) presentations. Note that over the past few decades it has become clear to clinicians and researchers that individuals can experience dementia and still retain their basic memory ability. These individuals are referred to as nonamnestic and show, for example, problems related to language performance such as finding the proper word, reduced spatial ability, or difficulty problem solving, which may include activities such as reasoning and judgment. Amnestic individuals are certainly more common and display "classic" deficits related to learning and the recall of new information. A probable AD diagnosis should not occur when clinicians have evidence of a stroke, which can also result in some of the above symptoms. In addition, it is suggested that a diagnosis of probable AD should not be applied to individuals who have experienced a history of small strokes, show disease involvement related to the other forms of dementia, or have an active neurological disease.[20]

Possible AD

A diagnosis of possible AD may be applied when an individual meets the core criteria as outlined, but the symptoms related to cognitive impairment are sudden or if it is difficult to determine when they started. As well, a possible AD designation may occur in cases where there is not an objective measure of cognitive difficulties, or in cases without a clear-cut sign that deficits are related to Alzheimer's disease. This means that if an individual has experienced a stroke or has another illness that makes it difficult to determine what is causing the onset of deficits, one may receive a diagnosis of possible AD. With the application of these new guidelines, individuals who previously met the criteria for possible AD may not meet them any more, and therefore will not receive this designation.[21]

It is important to keep in mind that, when evaluating or diagnosing either possible or probable AD, clinicians use a myriad of tests. This is because there is currently no single test that can give a definitive diagnosis of AD. Thus, an individual might undergo a number of laboratory tests, such as urinalysis, microscopy, or blood count to investigate the effects of anemia or infection. Serum electrolyte levels may be examined to investigate a possible metabolic disease, including liver function tests, and a thyroid panel may be used to rule out hypothyroidism. Serum vitamin B12 is also examined to rule out a deficiency (which is often related to memory deficits; however, note that serum tests may not be accurate enough for this type of evaluation and additional testing is required). Other tests examine neurosyphilis serology, urine toxicology, and serum toxicology.[22]

In addition, clinicians often will investigate deficits through the use of a number of radiology tools, such as X-ray, CT (computerized, or computed, tomography), SPECT (single photon emission computed tomography), PET (positron emission tomography), and MRI (magnetic resonance imaging). These tools are used to look for possible symptoms and to exclude other diseases that may be affecting the brain and brain tissue. Currently, MRI is able to detect brain tissue loss patterns typical of later stage AD. This tool can help distinguish AD cases from other types of dementia.[23] Research has shown that high-resolution imaging like MRI, fMRI (functional MRI), and especially PET can detect changes in brain tissue and brain chemistry. Past research shows that reported deficiencies can be observed within 94 percent accuracy when identifying reductions of fluorodeoxyglucose in AD patients over a period of time, which indicates an individual suffering from neurodegeneration.[24]

PROGRESSION OF AD

Providing a specific duration of time that any given individual will live with Alzheimer's disease is not possible; at best, one can give a ballpark figure. This is because the rate at which one individual progresses versus another can be quite different. One can read up on average rates online or in texts, but it is important to note that these are average rates and can fail to take into consideration several factors, such as when the individual was diagnosed, the involvement of other diseases, sex, and age at disease onset, to name a few.[25] General observations can be made about how individuals progress in the early stages as reflected by cognitive measurements. One suggestion is that quick progression, as shown by poor cognitive performance ability, can indicate illness at later stages.[26] Researchers have also suggested that biomarker measures, such as high levels of tau in one's cerebral spinal fluid (CSF), have been linked to a faster rate of cognitive decline in the latter stages of the illness.[27] Additional evidence has linked genetics and quicker deterioration to early-onset cases. Individuals with the familial form of AD have reported faster rates of decline; interestingly, these rates can also be influenced by one's level of both physical and cognitive health.[28] Thus, though someone can look up guidelines related to stage of illness and rates of progression, these values may prove unhelpful. Individuals may therefore not have a full understanding of the variations involved in personal AD progression. In fact, some research has suggested that the variability of individual progression is as large as the mean values of a specified stage (as measured via cognitive scores).[29] Therefore, one's rate of progression could be extended or decreased by several years based on numerous factors.

I could provide some general information related to the idea that if one is at this stage of the disease, then one has about this much time left. However, in doing so, I would risk depersonalizing the illness and possibly harm the efforts an individual is putting into fighting the progression of the disease. In addition, it is important to highlight that some of the current data we have on disease timelines is based on older patient information, which means that it doesn't factor in new interventions, including medications, cognitive training, and lifestyle changes. These have the ability to significantly alter the progression of the disease, as I have been pointing out throughout this book. Because of human nature, it is understandable that individuals afflicted with AD would want to know how much time they have, and answering with "that depends" is not acceptable to many. The point is that if this is the answer you or your loved one receives from your practitioners, this is not bad news. It really does depend on what mechanisms you are able to put in place. Having a plan of attack for some may significantly affect their disease progression, and as such, putting a timeline on this process may discourage rather than encourage action.

SEX AND AD

Engaging in an intimate sexual relationship with an individual afflicted with AD is viewed at times as both supportive (e.g., it helps reaffirm emotional ties) and on other occasions distressing (e.g., caregivers may worry about the level of consent). Individuals who view their ongoing sexual relationship as a source of support appear to do so as a way to deal with a sense of distance that can exist through the development and progression of AD. For many couples, sex is one of the last primary and positive aspects of their relationship that is "normal" and reaffirms their commitment to one another.[30] Disentangling the presence of AD in relation to other factors that affect sexual intimacy for couples is difficult. For example, one of the most influential markers in all our lives is that of stress. In the case of individuals caring for someone with AD, stress is a significant caregiver burden. When caregiver burden is examined, results indicate that as an individual's burden increases, engagement in sexual activities decreases. Specifically, studies note that couples dealing with AD have a significant reduction in sexual intercourse, with some research suggesting that it stops altogether.[31] If the caregiver burden increases as the illness progresses, then the subsequent result is a reduction in sexual activities, which is still observed when compared to couples of a similar age. In fact, one study finds that out of a sample of 162 individuals (average age 76.80 for the caregiver and 73.28 for the patient) only 27.9 percent of patients were able to stay engaged in sex without losing attention or arousal; these rates were similar for both men and women (as rated over a one-month time period). In addition, caregivers reported that when their loved one affected by AD did engage in sexual intimacy, only a third completed activity to the satisfaction of their partner.[32] This research clearly indicates that couples afflicted with AD still have a great interest in engaging in sexual activities. In fact, the majority of individuals want to maintain an intimate relationship with their loved one and often view it as a way to be supportive.[33] Note, however, that for females the loss of an emotional connection is linked to a reduction in their sexual satisfaction.[34] Therefore, even though health issues (normally occurring in men) are the primary reason for a lack of sexual intercourse in couples, the activity may still be tainted by a lack of the connection previously present. Interestingly, it is also noted that male caregivers report higher rates of sexual intercourse than the female caregivers. The belief here is that female caregivers are less focused on their own needs, and more focused on the core of the individual. However, for men it is suggested that their desire will continue in the face of minor changes in their partner, whereas women find this experience much more stressful.[35]

As just mentioned, men experience the majority of health concerns interfering with a couple's ability to engage in sexual intercourse. One of the primary problems receiving much attention in men is erectile dysfunction. Some researchers have reported that over 50 percent of men may experience erectile problems as a result of the onset of Alzheimer's disease. Interestingly, this study reported that this inability was not related to one's level of cognitive impairment, type of medication being used, or degree of depression. Thus, the researchers expected rates of erectile problems to be much lower, especially since other than the diagnosis of AD these individuals were fairly healthy.[36] There is no clear indication from this research why individuals will experience erectile dysfunction, but one suggestion is that this problem might be related to underlying brain pathways responsible for maintaining arousal. Additionally, being faced with such an illness and understanding its consequences can have a significant psychological impact. This psychological component will undoubtedly play a role in the desire to engage in sexual acts. One way to counter this problem, if it is truly based on a psychological issue, is for the couple to sit down and discuss concerns they have about the disease moving forward and their ability and desire to be intimate. Getting to the root of how the disease is affecting both of you and sharing your concerns will go a long way toward providing understanding and will improve the emotional and psychological components of your relationship.

In relation to sexual issues, one concern often cited by caregivers is that their significant other will engage in sexually inappropriate behavior. This worry is of great concern to caregivers particularly when they are out in public. They worry about the AD individual's decreased ability to censor comments or to refrain from sexually overt acts such as masturbation. It is difficult to ascertain where this worry may come from (perhaps word of mouth or small case reports); regardless, it is important to point out that current research suggests that such behavior is very rare. In fact, hypersexuality or talking to noncaregivers in sexual ways is rather limited, occurring in only about 7 percent of cases.[37] This rate is for cases where an individual has at some point said something the caregiver reports as inappropriate. On the other hand, caregivers may also find it difficult to deal with AD individuals because they can become sexual at times with what they perceive as inappropriate behavior. For instance, caregivers report AD individuals have trouble remembering that they engaged in sexual activity earlier that evening, or one minute they seem very interested in sex and at another not at all. These types of situations are very stressful for caregivers, and it is often reflected in the whole issue of sexual intimacy and AD.[38]

In reviewing the research for this topic, one of the key points often mentioned is the need for professionals to be proactive in discussing sexual relationships with couples experiencing dementia-related diseases. Health professionals agree that maintaining and accessing a sexual relationship is important to the couples' care. Because of the sensitive nature of this topic, many professionals leave it up to the couple to ask questions on sexual concerns. But if the health professional addresses this issue and communicates what is commonly observed on the sexual front (some of which is described above), it provides couples an opening to then ask questions or discuss any concerns they may be having. Having health professionals provide some structure to sexual conversation can improve ongoing care and ensure a more positive home environment, possibly reducing the need for early transfer to a long-term care facility.

A common misconception is that older couples and couples with AD are not sexually active or interested in sex. Thus, health professionals may think this topic does not need to be addressed.[39] However, it has been shown that sex is a very good way for couples to maintain a connection to one another and ensure the presence of intimacy. In addition, even if an individual has entered a long-term care facility, these institutions should be aware that it is important to provide the opportunity for couples to engage in sexual acts. Restricting a sexual relationship may affect the overall health of the couple and overall care.[40]

Ongoing research in this area is very important because the idea of what constitutes a couple has changed over the years, and soon these individuals will be seeking knowledge on how to handle sexuality and dementia. The creation of a body of knowledge that is accessible to all, and that promotes ongoing discussions of sexuality and dementia, will help couples understand they are not alone.

CHOLESTEROL AND AD

As noted previously, the APO E4 gene is linked to an increased risk of AD. E4 is often observed in the familial form of AD, and if your parents were carriers, you have a significantly increased risk of developing AD. This often results in a much earlier onset than sporadic AD. Recent research has shown that there is a metabolic relationship occurring between a gene called ABCA1 and APO E. This ABCA1 gene is believed to regulate APO E function through its "job" as a cellular cholesterol transporter. Outside the central nervous system, ABCA1 stimulates cholesterol transport via APOA-1, but within the central nervous system cholesterol is transported by APO E. APO E is important because it influences Aβ peptides, which facilitate the formation of amyloid plaques. Thus, the current theory is that if ABCA1 is overexpressed by a factor of six or more, it creates APO E that is lipid-enriched, resulting in the reduction of amyloidogenesis (the manufacturing of amyloid).[41] What this means is that at a basic level the production of plaques in the brain can be influenced by one's cholesterol system. This research is exciting because it suggests that a process can be designed to reduce the formation of amyloid plaques on the brain through genetic manipulation. Of course, researchers are just at the first stages of understanding all aspects of this relationship, including the mechanisms involved. But in light of this information, the goal now will be developing this as a treatment for certain causes of AD.

PREVENTING ALZHEIMER'S DISEASE

Can we prevent Alzheimer's disease? This is most likely the first and most important question you would have after reading most of this chapter, particularly if you or a friend or family member have the disease or you're predisposed to it. Therefore, let me say up front, the title of this section is somewhat misleading; there is no valid long-term evidence (yet) that indicates a definitive way to prevent the onset of Alzheimer's disease. However, what I can say is that there are currently many researchers and research centers interested in developing preventative programs for individuals who have or might acquire Alzheimer's disease. I will review some of these initiatives to demonstrate the important implications of this research.

Immunotherapy

Recent evidence reported by Norman Relkin and his colleagues at the Weill Cornell Medical College in New York suggests that it may be possible to treat AD using an immunotherapy program.[42] The highlight of this program was the stabilization of AD symptoms over a three-year period, which included measures of cognitive performance and quality of life. This is the first treatment program to show consistent, long-term cognitive stabilization. Individuals in the full three-year treatment program received intravenous immunoglobulin (IVIG) at a rate of 0.4g/kg every two weeks. IVIG is a "blood cocktail" that includes concentrated levels of antibodies taken from the blood plasma of one thousand or more individuals. Historically, this type of treatment is used for individuals who have immune deficiencies or antibody production problems. It is also helpful in cases where individuals have experienced sudden infection onset. Individuals tolerated this therapy well, and all participants were in the mild to moderate stages of the disease. If there is a drawback to this study, it is that there were only sixteen patients that completed the full-term program. Though numbers are low, a fact acknowledged by the authors, the results clearly show that this group substantially outperformed controls. In addition, individuals who switched from the placebo group to the treatment group showed gains in previously noted performance deficit areas. These results look quite promising, but it is very early in this research program. Not until a larger group is evaluated, over a longer period of time, will researchers be able to understand the precise benefits of this treatment. These concerns aside, this is excellent news, and this type of therapy may be very important in the years to come.

Anti-Amyloid Treatment

As mentioned previously, one of the major processes involved in Alzheimer's disease is the buildup of amyloid plaque in the brain. Researchers have suggested that if this buildup could be slowed or stopped, the outlook for AD patients would be dramatically improved. A group led by Reisa Sperling of the Harvard Medical School and Women's Hospital in Boston has been working on the development of an anti-amyloid treatment.[43] This treatment will likely use a monoclonal antibody (which means that the immune system can be triggered to target certain cells or proteins for destruction, such as beta-amyloid). The goal for this research group is to target individuals with the predisposition (the genetic form E4) to AD, and then to start them on therapy prior to onset. The hope is that this type of treatment will prevent the development of amyloid or, if already in progress, slow its development. Of course, outright prevention would be monumental because damage as a result of beta-amyloid is one of the main concerns related to AD. If this could be silenced, the outlook for affected individuals would be excellent. Even slowing this progression significantly would be of great benefit since the familial form of AD often begins much earlier and progresses much quicker. Thus, developing a way to affect this progression for these individuals would be considerable. Currently, this type of therapy is under development, and as such, success is not known. In addition, it is important to note that this therapy is designed to affect amyloid, and therefore the ongoing concern of tau will still be present. Therefore, there is no guarantee that the disease will not continue to progress in the tau form.

The Alzheimer's Prevention Initiative

A group of researchers led by Eric Reiman, who is from the Banner Alzheimer's Institute in Phoenix, Arizona, is developing a prevention program for individuals genetically at risk for developing AD. Research has suggested that changes in the brain of individuals who will exhibit AD occur many years prior to disease onset. The suggestion from this group, in fact, is that brain changes are detectable up to fifteen years before behavioral symptoms begin to appear.[44] Individuals who show these early changes in their brain are identified as having presymptomatic Alzheimer's disease. The researchers believe the best way to combat AD is to treat it before it starts. The goal is to use neuroimaging evidence and other methods (e.g., cerebral spinal fluids, cognitive measures) to identify and track changes in individuals as therapies such as gene modifying treatments and amyloid reduction are applied. Tracking changes through specific biomarkers will provide a level of detail on the progression and development of the disease unlike any seen before. Thus, we will have greater insight into how the disease develops and possibly identify ways to change its course.

Though I have highlighted only three major projects in progress, this is by no means an exhaustive list of those underway. The progress, however, is very encouraging, and the goal of either eliminating this disease or providing a way to manage it seems achievable in the not too distant future. The evidence and research currently underway on Alzheimer's disease is some of the most promising in recent years. The largest threat to achieving a cure could be the reduction of funding to support such programs. Thus, it is important for us all to ensure our nation's health funding is meeting the needs of these programs.

7

CAN COGNITIVE TRAINING AFFECT THE COURSE OF AGING AND DISEASE?

After reading this chapter, you should be able to answer the following questions:

Can video games help my brain as I age?

Is there any point to cognitive training after I have been diagnosed with a cognitive impairment?

Are there any costs or benefits in using cognitive training programs?

GAMING/TRAINING PROGRAMS

There is a new, emerging market of computerized brain training websites developed specifically to help individuals exercise, enhance, and improve their brain. These sites vary and offer different exercises, but to a certain extent they all offer an opportunity for individuals to exercise their brain, with the overall goal of improving everyday performance on tasks such as attention, memory, and visuospatial ability. The big question of course is, do these activities really work? Can I have a better and healthier brain by engaging in these online tasks? Let's review some of the background research, beyond website testimonials or promotional commercials, to see whether programs such as these really make a difference.

As a society, we have evolved by integrating ourselves with technology, although the level of integration varies depending on the individual. The virtues of gaming have been rather limited until recent years, and "gamers" themselves have often come under attack for spending too much time doing something looked upon as offering little benefit to society. However, times are changing, and some good examples have been provided of why gaming may be good. One such example comes from the medical field, where they have asked the question, is there a positive to medical students playing video games? Well, in fact, there is. A study in 2011 showed that medical students who engaged in a minimum of seven hours per week of video gaming demonstrated significantly better psychomotor skills. These authors believe improved psychomotor skills are advantageous to careers in surgery and that gaming activities translate to useful skills for the operating room.[1] A literature review on this very topic also concluded that certain surgical skills were improved, in addition to overall performance on psychomotor tasks, as a result of playing video games.[2] In addition, evidence currently suggests that gamers hold a distinct advantage in basic cognitive skills (e.g., tracking objects, visual short-term memory, task switching).[3] The extent of this "brain advantage," particularly in varying ages, is not yet fully understood, but there are ongoing efforts to evaluate it.

I have offered up these initial examples to dispel the myth that gaming is all bad. In fact, the teenager next door who plays games all night might be the one operating on you ten years from now. By pointing out some positive attributes of gaming, I am simply trying to help you understand that engaging in activities via a computer or game system may hold some previously unthought-of benefits.

Though there are some basic highlighted benefits of gaming in general, for aging individuals it is not these general benefits people are after, but the specific benefits. If you take time to engage in a task, you want to know why, and if, it works. These, of course, are very valid questions.

Before providing some of the evidence, I should first point out that, not surprisingly, the effects of video gaming on older people have not been extensively examined, although they have certainly gained attention in the past few years for a number of reasons. One of these reasons is that the generation who grew up with home gaming systems is now of the age where they are researchers, and they are curious about the effects of the activities they have engaged in for a lifetime and how they might be used for health benefits. In addition to this, because of our rapidly aging population, both aging individuals and health-care professionals are trying to find new ways to supplement dwindling services, information, and attention.

Do Video Game Activities Work for an Aging Individual?

The answer is yes! Video games have been shown to be effective in assisting aging individuals improve a number of skills, yet what is of greater interest is how these games help and what skills they improve. Initially, researchers were interested in examining if playing basic "original" games (e.g., *Donkey Kong*, *Pac-Man*, *Tetris*) would lead to general, overall better cognitive performance. These initial studies showed what specific improvements could be observed by playing one of the "original" games. For example, one study found that aging individuals (between the ages of fifty-seven and eighty-three) playing *Donkey Kong* and *Pac-Man* saw improvements in their choice response times, meaning they got faster at tasks where they were required to decide quickly on the correct response.[4] Thus, in this case, aging individuals' game playing practices generalized to tasks requiring quick judgment and selection. Further examination in this area has also shown that aging individuals (from sixty-nine to ninety) playing the game *Super Tetris* had substantially improved their reaction time and in some cases their sense of well-being. However, in regards to *Super Tetris*, it is important to note that the authors indicate that weaker effects were observed on cognitive performance measures, suggesting that gains are specific to the type of task being undertaken.[5] Though this might seem to be a negative, it can also provide insight into how these tasks can be used. For example, we know one can become generally quicker on visually guided motor control tasks, which is an excellent bonus, particularly in the face of advanced aging.

These results are fantastic because they show that improvement occurs on some level in the aging brain. Researchers wondered if more complex games or a combination of games could be used to improve more complex cognitive processes, such as memory, reasoning, and planning abilities (i.e., frontal lobe tasks). In recent years, researchers set out to examine this question. For example, one study used a set of seven video games chosen for their presumed ability to improve concentration, processing speed, procedural tasks, and working memory.[6] Another study chose a game that provided real-time feedback and was highly strategic, requiring constant attention to various components of game play and the implementation of an overall strategy.[7] Other researchers focused on a game they believed tapped into "executive control" (e.g., divided attention, visual scanning, and working memory), which they found more effective in creating a transfer to everyday cognitive skills.[8] What these studies have in common is that they all report, at some level, improved performance in aging populations on cognitive tasks such as working memory, visual short-term memory, task switching, reasoning, and quality of life. This list of benefits is most promising and is encouraged by increased examination of the use of complex games to help alter our cognitive processes. However, these tasks are presented in strict settings with strict controls, and participant gamers are excited and no doubt trying to provide their best each and every time. Thus, if this training seems desirable to you, keep in mind that undivided attention is very important to achieving these benefits.

One might think, "Great, this might be a very helpful component in keeping me on top of my game as I age. But what happens if I have a brain that is under attack from cognitive disease? Is there anything I can do to help my brain then?" Well, as it just so happens, there are current studies underway to help us understand what we can do if we have been afflicted with a neurodegenerative disease such as Alzheimer's.

GAMING/TRAINING AND ALZHEIMER'S DISEASE

Individuals afflicted with Alzheimer's disease (AD) have historically thought that there was not much that could be done and that medication to help combat this assault on their brain was really the only option. This can be extremely problematic for individuals who are unable for a variety of reasons to take certain medications. However, in recent years researchers have found that medication is not the only option. Cognitive training for AD patients is a relatively new area of research, and as recently as 2004 it was reported that no empirically validated cognitive treatment procedures existed for AD.[9] However, more recent studies have reported that cognitive training, in addition to cholinesterase inhibitors (medication), may be effective in enhancing or stabilizing cognition in mild AD. For example, one study using an eight-week computer-based program consisting of two blocks of sixteen sessions of various cognitive exercises demonstrated that mildly affected AD patients on stable doses of cholinesterase inhibitors significantly improved on tests of global cognition (MMSE score), verbal production, and executive functioning.[10] Additionally, a single-blind randomized pilot study comparing the addition of psychostimulation or cognitive stimulation to cholinesterase inhibitors in mild AD patients revealed improved scores on tests of global cognition, which were maintained until the study ended at twenty-four weeks.[11] Similarly, mild AD patients on a stable dose of cholinesterase inhibitors benefited from a cognitive rehabilitative intervention, demonstrating improvements in orientation, learning of face-name associations, speed of processing, and specific functional activities such as making change for a purchase. These training effects were maintained over the three-month period without any further maintenance sessions.[12]

Other studies have shown improvements in cognition and in activities of daily living (ADL), including positive changes in behavioral disturbances and caregiver stress. Researchers who used exercises aimed at rehabilitation of memory and ADLs in patients on stable doses of cholinesterase inhibitors saw significant improvements on ADLs and a small improvement in memory after a fourteen-week training program. Patients with mild to moderate AD or mild cognitive impairment on cholinesterase inhibitors, who received a cognitive-motor intervention, maintained cognitive status at six months and maintained or improved their affective status at one year relative to controls.[13]

One of the primary take-home messages from these studies is that computer-based intervention targeting individuals afflicted with AD, a disease previously thought unresponsive to nonmeditative intervention, can be effective. Thus, the goal now for many researchers is to understand the subtleties of such programs, why certain strategies are more effective than others and which areas of the brain should be targeted.

When it comes to targeting brain regions, trying to go head-on at the illness may not be very beneficial and can cause frustration for both the caregiver and the participant. Going head-on at the illness means, for example, targeting memory (if one has memory issues) on a daily basis, using a focused strategy to effect change and increase memory. For example, this might involve giving a list of ten words to an AD individual to read over each morning for thirty minutes, then taking the list away and asking him or her what those tens words were. As you can imagine, for an AD individual, this task will become very difficult and very frustrating. Remembering anything for any duration of time, especially unrelated words through a short-term memory task, will undoubtedly be difficult to complete. However, if every morning you give the AD individual a game to play that asks them to arrange shapes or find their way through a maze, the task will most likely not be as difficult and you will avoid a head-on collision with the disease (if memory is the primary concern). The goal of course is to increase overall performance, including memory, through access of other brain regions, which in turn can help stimulate affected areas via indirect routes.

There are, of course, numerous brain regions that work in collaboration every day in an effort to perform various tasks. Cutting-edge research examining the physiological structure of the nervous system has recently shown that one's brain has significant connections among its various regions. In fact, the structural integrity of a bundle of nerve fibers (the inferior longitudinal fasciculus, inferior occipitofrontal fasciculus, cingulate cortex, and posterior thalamic radiation) with connections between the parietal (i.e., action area), frontal (i.e., planning and organizing) and temporal (i.e., memory) brain regions is noted to be important in maintaining overall brain functioning. Research indicates that damage to these bundles of fibers in, say, the parietal areas could affect projections to regions such as the temporal.[14] Thus, I suggest that if these regional connections can be weakened by disease or trauma (e.g., traumatic brain injury), then strengthening one area may help others, or at the very least generate better connectivity. Though there is currently no definitive proof that this in fact happens, further research in the years to come might shed some light on this topic.

In conclusion, one might ask, should I incorporate video or mental games into my everyday efforts to maintain a healthy brain? Well, I believe the question is not so much should you, as how much, and in what ways. I believe there is a definitive answer to this question, and though some websites suggest that you can identify a weak area—which is true—it may not be the area that is of greatest concern, and targeting it may not help you maintain overall health. Therefore, the best advice is to alter your activities on an ongoing basis and exercise your whole brain, not just parts of it.

COGNITIVE TRAINING AND ALZHEIMER'S DISEASE NEUROPATHOLOGY

As evident from its classification, a neurodegenerative condition such as AD is a progressive and debilitating condition. However, despite this designation, the potential for cognitive plasticity is still present. In fact, evidence indicates that cognitive plasticity (i.e., the ability of the brain to adapt) can be observed in early AD. Research on AD patients has demonstrated greater activation in brain regions supporting memory and execution activities, indicating that the damaged brain is working harder.[15] In support of this, pathological research has noted that increases can be seen in synaptic contrast size.[16] Thus, the theory is that early stage AD creates an environment where the brain is attempting to compensate for deficits by increasing synaptic size and activity. Inducing changes in brain processes allows one to handle the onset of AD, but only for variable amounts of time. Not assisting with this process, in my opinion, means AD can progress more quickly, especially in certain individuals who are ill prepared to adapt to new challenges or changes in brain chemistry and structure. Evidence suggests that nonpharmacological adjunctive interventions such as cognitive stimulation activities, in conjunction with medication, can enhance one's abilities beyond what can be observed in just taking medication alone.[17]

COGNITIVE TRAINING AND AD

Rehabilitative procedures for AD patients are a relatively new area of research, and by no means is there expansive literature on this topic. A large review of the research in 2006 yielded nineteen solid studies (where proper protocol was followed and proper controls were put in place) focusing on cognitive training for individuals experiencing AD.[18] Interestingly, on average there were only sixteen subjects per study, suggesting that cognitive training among this population group has by no means been studied on a large scale. Overall, cognitive training does appear to provide some benefit, but what is causing this benefit is up for interpretation. It could be merely that the individual is routinely engaged in tasks with another individual, and it is this ongoing attention that helps improve mood and attention, keeping the individual generally mentally active. It could also be that restorative strategies (which work around the deficit but focus on keeping the brain active), as opposed to compensatory strategies (which try to fix a specific deficit), are more beneficial.

Additional research has indicated that when individuals with AD are provided opportunities to engage in cognitive training or cognitive rehabilitation programs, significant improvements occur. Specifically, one procedure showed cognitive improvement through the use of a computer-based program task, with improvements in memory (short term and long term), perception, and attention. In addition, studies of mild cognitive impairment (MCI) patients showed significant increases in working memory and psychomotor learning (understanding where to move when requested). Overall, significant improvements were observed on the Mini Mental Status Exam (MMSE), in verbal fluency, and on planning and organizing tasks.[19] One program addressed the effectiveness of using a specified cognitive stimulation procedure versus a more global approach. Results showed that global stimulation, rather than specific cognitive procedures, is more successful (similar to what is reported above), as evidenced by improvements in verbal fluency, behavioral disturbances, and caregiver stress.[20] Other approaches suggest that the most effective measure to slow the progression of AD is through the combination of cognitive training procedures and pharmacological treatments (e.g., cholinesterase inhibitors).[21] Mildly impaired AD patients on cholinesterase inhibitors exhibited improved performance on orientation, learning of face-name associations, speed of processing, and specific functional abilities. This group also benefited from weekly stimulation of their memories and language ability, which in turn improved cognitive functioning and activities of daily living.

Functional skills training was associated with successful maintenance of cognitive gains over a three-month interval. Two primary points noted by researchers is that functional training that more closely resembled real-world situations resulted in the greatest benefit to patients, and improved performance on these functional tests may be a direct result of visuomotor training. Thus, this study noted the importance of visuomotor processing in providing a positive effect on cognitive improvement for AD patients.[22] This suggests that future research needs to explore this type of design to determine the overreaching effects.

Although many of the studies presented here demonstrate general cognitive improvement, the results should be tempered by the fact that these improvements are not observed in all domains or in all studies, especially when individuals have reached a more advanced stage of moderate to severe impairment. Although cognitive gains were not observed in all patients, their performance in some cases remained at a relatively stable level, providing optimism that the neurodegenerative disease was encountering resistance of some kind.

Three major points can be drawn from this review of AD and cognitive training. One is that this process demonstrates success, evidenced by substantial cognitive change on many levels. Second, since these substantial changes can be observed, the opportunity exists to address this disease on different levels. Finally, training initiatives should be extended to address the more global impairments associated with AD. To date, cognitive training programs have been mainly pilot applications for AD patients. Thus, there has been limited focus on the stimulation of various brain regions—for example, the parietal region, which has had limited examination even though considerable deficits can be observed, especially in visually guided motor tasks.[23] Thus, to deal with deficits in visuomotor/visuospatial (e.g., parietal lobe activities) performance and promote global rehabilitation (noted to affect general cognitive decline), designing training procedures to engage the parietal networks could be a viable option in rehabilitating a region substantially affected by the progression of AD.[24] These procedures could improve the quality of life for many individuals, and further investigation is needed.

THE COST-EFFECTIVENESS OF COGNITIVE STIMULATION THERAPY

First and foremost, when one reads the term *cost-effectiveness*, one thinks about how much money can be saved. But cost-effectiveness needs to be examined on a larger scale; governments need to be aware that a little bit of money up front could potentially protect their citizens from a more serious and drastic decline when faced with a dementia-related illness. On a personal front, cost-effectiveness can also refer to the cost of maintaining one's level of ability for as long as possible, and to "retain oneself" is of such importance that individuals need to be aware of the cost of doing nothing.

The overall picture is this: research on cognitive stimulation therapy (CST) demonstrates its capacity to be a cost-effective option for the treatment of AD. Quality of life and cognition improvements can be observed with the introduction of cognitive stimulation therapy. CST improvements are more beneficial when compared to standard treatments.[25] This research also highlights the importance of using cognitive therapy techniques to address dementia-related illnesses and the advantages that can be gained with the application of straightforward cognitive programs within these populations. To further examine these interventions, the next section will give an understanding of the true monetary and human costs associated with this type of activity.

CST'S MONETARY AND HUMAN COSTS

The cost breakdown of how effective CST programs are or can be has received relatively limited examination since there is no one way to evaluate these types of programs. Deciding on what to measure, and how to measure it, influences the cost greatly. In addition, because of these inconsistencies, trying to make direct comparisons across different studies can prove difficult. However, despite these issues, great strides have been taken to try to pin down costs associated with CST.

A study in 2006 examined the cost-effectiveness of CST in the UK in an effort to understand the willingness to pay for cognitive change. The authors mapped things such as the cost of achieving a one-point increase on a cognitive scale such as the MMSE, which was put at £102.00 ($156.00 USD). For the quality of life scale, a one-point change cost £22.82 ($36.00 USD). These amounts, particularly the second, were deemed relatively low since families indicated that they would pay on average £100.00 ($154.00 USD) for effective change. These authors noted that a one-point decline in the MMSE score for an individual just taking medication (donepezil) was equated to £56.00 ($86.00 USD) of the direct cost to health and social care. This number excludes the costs of medication and institutionalization, which of course would be significant. Thus, they suggest that CST could be of greater value monetarily and would be far superior to relying on medication only for treatment.

Finally, they wondered if the factor affecting this change in the CST groups could be related to the social component of CST and not the intervention itself. However, the researchers examined control data for social-only groups and determined that the difference was in fact due to CST and not just the social interaction.[26] Though this research focused primarily on monetary concerns, I think it would be safe to say that an increase in one's quality of life scores, rather than seeing a continual decrease, is a significant gain for both the individuals and their families, thus reducing the "human cost" as well.

Additional studies not examining either of these costs directly have nevertheless shown that cognitive programs are successful in creating cognitive change. On average, a yearly decrease of 1.8 to 4.2 points in the MMSE score is typical for an AD patient.[27] Given this understanding, several researchers have demonstrated that cognitive therapy programs can counteract this decline (note that no movement in scores at all would in fact be a gain with this disease). Research suggests that the longer and more often one engages in cognitive training programs, the greater the effect they have on staving off significant cognitive decline and increasing the time individuals are able to stay at home.[28] It has also been suggested that maintenance (ongoing cognitive activities) is essential for individuals with AD. Thus, cognitive programs are good opportunities to effect immediate change; however, research has also suggested that these programs need to have periods of ongoing activity to help maintain cognitive gains. If they do not, individuals can deteriorate as early as twenty-three weeks after the cognitive intervention.

Researchers have also examined interventions related to managing AD and dementia patients. Many facilities report issues related to agitation, behavioral disturbances, and physical injuries (e.g., falls). One study in 2012 noted that with the application of a behavior management program, which was a combination therapy program that included elements of music, memory props, and tailored DVDs related to comfort and stimulation, resulted in individuals increasing their engagement with the staff and reducing their agitation levels, which in turn reduced time spent handling upset residents and freed staff up to engage in better care. In addition, these researchers noted that falls were reduced by 32.5 percent during the first six months of this study.[29] It is important to note that this program used a combination of therapies for behavior management, including stimulation activities. Though many of these results are observational only, I think it ties in well with the theory that cognitive stimulation activities have a multitude of benefits and can be easily applied and implemented in various settings.

Though I have not listed any direct cost related to these programs, you can be assured that maintaining an individual in a community and at home is, on a personal level, less stressful for the individual and for family members as well. Of course, direct caregivers are an exception, since they experience significant amounts of stress at times dealing with their loved one, and having to choose a long-term placement (if available and one can afford it) is a very difficult decision. Thus, having cognitive training programs in place that are accessible, ongoing, and utilized effectively by the community could be cost-effective, especially when you look at the figures involved in treating individuals as we have in the past.

Data from U.S. Alzheimer's Society suggest that if we can delay long-term nursing home care by one month, one billion dollars a year could be saved.[30] In addition, a report from the Alzheimer's Society of Ontario, Canada, noted that by promoting prevention programs (which includes cognitive programs), as much as eleven billion dollars could be saved over the next decade, including a reduction of sixty-three thousand new cases of AD each year.[31] Prevention programs and activities such as the ones discussed in this book can help delay the onset of dementia. In addition to these significant cost savings, which hopefully do not go unnoticed by governments and communities, there is the personal cost savings. If this were happening to you or your loved one, what would you give to get back five years, or even one year, of good brain health? What would that be worth? What would it be worth to maintain one's autonomy or sense of self for just an extra six months? Programs such as these may add years of good cognitive health, and to many this would be priceless. Thus, the "human cost" is incalculable and should never be taken for granted.

8

COGNITIVE ENHANCEMENTS

After reading this chapter, you should be able to answer the following questions:

Are there medications available that can affect my cognitive performance?

Is there a prescription for Alzheimer's disease?

What is the role of neurotransmitters?

Cognitive enhancements is a term used for pharmacological interventions to boost cognitive performance, and it is a term that will increase in familiarity in the years to come. In regard to aging and age-related degeneration, most cognitive enhancement medications have been developed to combat cognitive decline related to dementia-related disturbances, mainly for individuals with possible or probable Alzheimer's disease. I will discuss in detail in this chapter medications that are commonly used for the treatment of dementia-related decline. However, before I provide this review, I want to talk in general about the rise of cognitive enhancement drugs, how they are currently being used, and how they might be used in the future.

In recent years, there have been increasing reports of the use of neuroenhancers (i.e., "smart drugs"), showing that in some circles they have been gaining in popularity. Though the goal of neural enhancement is medications that can alter the course of specific cognitive impairments, as with many things in our society, segments of the population will undoubtedly come up with alternative ways to use such resources. One novel approach has been to evaluate if these same types of drugs can improve normal cognitive performance.

Cognition, or thought processes, often gets boiled down to a few things, such as planning, memory retrieval, and decision making, and as such it is examined in relation to one's errorless performance, speed of processing, and judgment ability. Though researchers are great at applying arbitrary separation between these abilities and then measuring performance via specific output scales, the truth is that these measurements fall well short of defining "innate" cognitive processing. In fact, though neuroscience has made great advances, we actually still do not know much about neurobiology as it relates to characteristics of cognitive networks.[1] Despite these shortcomings, scientists have pushed forward by examining the drugs known as cognitive enhancers, called this because of the effects they have on an individual's physiological state. By "physiological state" I mean a change, for instance, in an individual's arousal level (e.g., attention).

The "list of drugs potentially enhancing memory is rather long and includes drugs acting on neurotransmitters, on hormones, on transduction systems and brain perfusion and metabolism."[2] One of the main concerns with any drug is determining its effects on one set of desired outcomes ("brain gains") at the expense of other physiological processes. For example, differences in attention are commonly observed with the use of a drug such as methylphenidate (Ritalin) in an effort to determine performance on and off the medication. Ritalin, though commonly prescribed to individuals experiencing attentional disorders, has also been examined for its effects on normally functioning individuals. Initially, it was thought that if this drug can correct attentional issues in "dysfunctioning" brains, then it could possibly create a heightened ability in a "normal" brain. In fact, many media sources have reported that university students use Ritalin to improve "memory recall" and "boost brain power," with little attention paid to its actual effect in retaining information.[3] Though certain short-term effects on attention and arousal appear beneficial for users of Ritalin, researchers suggest that after twenty-four hours these effects can dissipate. Also, high concentrations can actually induce impairment, rather than improve performance. However, results vary widely, and it often depends on the individual and the situation.[4] In summary, Ritalin has generally not been very successful for enhancing "brain power" in regard to long-term learning, and extensive nonprescription use might create an impairment.

Another drug recently examined is modafinil (Provigil). Around for about twenty years, it was initially marketed for excessive sleepiness. However, as with Ritalin, modafinil has been examined to determine if it can improve mental performance in normally functioning individuals. Current reports have suggested that, at best, it has selective ability to improve some areas related to attention, and some mild effects have been noted in working memory. Thus, similar to Ritalin, this drug can affect attention, most likely due to increased arousal, resulting in some improvement in working memory.[5]

The larger question in relation to these drugs is if cognition is affected or altered. Research to date suggests that only changes in physiology occur, and this type of medication does not seem to offer long-term or markedly large changes in one's intelligence. If it did, I'm certain it would be in much greater demand, and "we the public" would have heard much more about these miraculous effects.

So this leaves a lingering question: are there drugs in the works that can alter long-term cognition for individuals with average ability? The quick answer is yes. Researchers are currently examining the properties of several drugs, some of which are quite common (e.g., caffeine and nicotine) and some not so common (e.g., ampakine). All drugs thought to have cognitive-enhancing properties should be examined to see if long-term performance and improved memory ability can be achieved, which would provide us with a better understanding of their effects on cognitive ability.

Ampakine is a drug identified to affect AMPA-type glutamate neuro-receptors (meaning it increases energy levels at certain sites in the brain). One study recently examined if rats given the drug could increase their performance on complex behavioral tasks. What researchers found was that rats actually exceeded their expected ability, and the effects of the drug lasted long after use, indicating complex cognitive processes were affected.[6] Whether this ability can be observed in humans is yet to be determined, but assuredly several studies are underway to examine ways we can expand our performance beyond its predetermined level. Current drugs under investigation include piracetam, aniracetam, nimodipine, idebenone, mirtazapine, oxiracetam, and nefiracetam, to name a few. These drugs are known to have varying effects on memory and attention and continue to be examined in relation to "off label" (not as directed) use. In addition to experiments with these manufactured drugs, there has also been a boom in nutritional products that might increase cognitive ability the natural way, though the evidence is not clear. This industry alone has reached a billion dollars annually in the United States.[7]

Why is there so much interest in this area of research right now? One reason could be that, as a "global village," we are increasingly exposed, or some might say overexposed, to significant amounts of information. Some might believe the best way to handle this "hyper-technological age" is through the use of cognitive-enhancing materials. If I want to get ahead and stay up-to-date with all this information, one way I may be able to help myself is by increasing my brain capacity. When you can go into any electronics store and pick up an external terabyte hard drive, you know we are in an age where information is dominant. To keep up with this increase, many are seeking ways to enhance their minds, explaining the billion dollars spent annually in the United States alone, despite some mixed results. Another explanation could be our aging workforce. Many individuals currently are working into their retirement years and might be looking for that little extra help to maintain or enhance their own personal performance. In addition, people are simply living longer, and cognitive diseases that may not have been an issue years ago (because higher mortality rates at earlier ages reduced the number of elderly worldwide) are becoming more apparent, simply by the shear number of individuals faced with an aging brain. One might argue that aging generations are also better informed on their options as they move into their later years. Whatever the reasons may be, there is a great interest in maintaining one's cognitive ability, and rightly so!

Though it is apparent that maintaining cognitive vivacity is of great importance to our world's normal aging population, it is also of great importance to individuals experiencing cognitive difficulties. Alzheimer's disease has been the poster child for cognitive impairment, and as a result much research has gone into examining ways to alter its progression. One of the ways researchers have been trying to do this is through the medications that affect the transmission of information within the brain. These medications do not directly combat the disease but instead use alternative means to keep the brain as active as possible and provide it assistance by increasing the "tools" available to the individual. I will describe some of the most recognized medications currently used and prescribed below.

NEUROTRANSMITTERS (BRAIN MESSENGERS)

Before I describe current medication designed to combat the effects of cognitive impairment, I would like to provide some information about neurotransmitters and their role in your brain's ability to send messages. The brain is made up of around eighty-six billion neurons, each of which makes connections with other neurons in your brain.[8] In order to work with one another, they need to send and receive information. This occurs by sending special messengers called neurotransmitters across the small gap (known as a synapse) between the cells. In some cases, the goal is to excite the neuron into generating an action (e.g., pay attention to these directions); in others, to inhibit an action (e.g., don't drop your coffee even though it is hot). Thus, the number and type of neurotransmitters being sent across the synapse will depend on the ability of the neuron to act. Current medications for Alzheimer's disease focus on altering the amount and type of neurotransmitters available in the synapse junction, and this subsequently affects the ability of the neuron. Such medications primarily increase two types of neurotransmitters: acetylcholine and glutamate. The goal is to increase the amount of acetylcholine and glutamate available in the synapses, which helps facilitate messages being sent and received between neurons. However, it is important to keep in mind that in a neurodegenerative condition such as Alzheimer's disease, this process will only be beneficial for a certain amount of time, and results can vary widely based on the individual. Despite this, these medications can be very effective for certain durations of time, and in some cases I have seen individuals regain lost abilities, though not permanently.

When an individual receives a diagnosis of possible or probable AD, one of the first questions families often have is, what can we do? It is important to understand that a disease such as Alzheimer's cannot be eradicated by a vaccination or reversed by medications—yet! However, medications can treat the symptoms of Alzheimer's disease. The goal, therefore, is to give these individuals the ability to maintain cognitive ability for as long as possible through the alteration of their "brain resources."

PRIMARY MEDICATIONS USED TO TREAT ALZHEIMER'S DISEASE

Common medication treatments for Alzheimer's disease in North America are the following: Aricept (donepezil), Exelon (rivastigmine), Reminyl (galantamine hydrobromide), Ebixa or Namenda (memantine hydrochloride), and Cognex (tacrine). Note that all information about medications is available at the manufacturers' websites (including updates). The following information about medications was retrieved from the Alzheimer's Societies: United States, Canada, and the United Kingdom (http://www.alzheimer.ca/en/Living-with-dementia/Treatment-options/Drugs-approved-for-Alzheimers-disease [Alzheimer's Society Canada]; http://www.alz.org/research/science/alzheimers_disease_treatments.asp#approved [Alzheimer's Society U.S.]; http://www.alzheimers.org.uk/site/scripts/documents_info.php?documentID=147 [Alzheimer's Society U.K.]

Aricept

Aricept (donepezil): Intended for use with mild to moderate AD (5 mg white tablets; after four to six weeks, 10 mg yellow tablets all contain donepezil hydrochloride).

Aricept is a "cholinesterase inhibitor." It is designed to inhibit acetylcholinesterase, the enzyme responsible for breaking down acetylcholine. AD is noted to reduce the amount of acetylcholine, creating disruption in learning and memory. The subsequent effect of Aricept is that it increases the amount of acetylcholine, thereby increasing the potential for neuron transmission and improving sensitivity in receptor regions. Thus, the role of Aricept is to minimize the effects of disease progression.

Before taking Aricept, notify your physician if any of these conditions exist: if you are allergic to donepezil hydrochloride or piperidine derivatives such as Mycobutin (rifabutin), Ritalin (methylphenidate), Akineton (biperiden HCI), Artane (trihexyphenidyl HCI), Bupivacaine

HCI, and Paxil (paroxetine HCI); if you have a condition affecting your heart (rhythm disorder) or your lungs (asthma); if you have had seizures; if you have had fainting spells; and if you have a history of peptic ulcers or have an increased risk of developing ulcers (for example, if you are taking nonsteroidal anti-inflammatory drugs [NSAIDs] or high doses of acetylsalicylic acid [ASA/Aspirin]), or have an enlarged prostate. Aricept should not be used if you are pregnant or breastfeeding.

Exelon

Exelon (rivastigmine): Intended for use with mild to moderate AD (3–6 mg twice daily; 12 mg daily often prescribed).

Exelon is another cholinesterase inhibitor. It targets the cholinesterase enzyme that is normally broken down by acetylcholine. As with Aricept, the goal of Exelon is to increase the amount of acetylcholine available to the brain. Exelon facilitates greater interaction between nerve cells and heightens sensitivity in receptors, helping with cognition and memory processes.

Before taking Exelon, notify your physician if any of these conditions exist: any conditions affecting your heart or lungs; if you have seizures; if you have had fainting spells; and if you have a history of peptic ulcers or have increased risk of developing ulcers (for example, if you are taking nonsteroidal anti-inflammatory drugs [NSAIDs] or high doses of acetylsalicylic acid [ASA/Aspirin]).

Reminyl

Reminyl (Razadyne in the United States) (galantamine hydrobromide): Intended for use with mild to moderate AD (extended-release tablet taken once daily; 8–24 mg often prescribed; 8 mg white capsule, 16 mg pink capsule, 24 mg caramel opaque capsules).

Reminyl is another cholinesterase inhibitor designed to treat symptoms of AD. Galantamine is designed to prevent acetylcholinesterase (the process involved in breaking down acetylcholine compound). Galantamine also increases the activity of the acetylcholine present in the brain. Thus, as with the others, it is designed to help cognitive functions, such as thinking and problem solving.

Before taking Reminyl, notify your physician if any of these conditions exist: if you have a heart disorder, liver problems, kidney problems, stomach ulcer or a history of ulcer, acute abdominal pain, disorders of the nervous system (like epilepsy), respiratory diseases that interfere with breathing (like asthma), a recent operation on the stomach or bladder, or difficulties in passing urine; if you have an increased risk of developing ulcers (for example, if you are currently using nonsteroidal anti-inflammatory drugs [NSAIDs] or high doses of acetylsalicylic acid [ASA/Aspirin]) or fungal infections, or if you are a woman of childbearing age, pregnant, possibly pregnant, or a nursing mother.

Exiba

Ebixa or Namenda (memantine hydrochloride): Intended for use with moderate to severe AD (Ebixa starts at 5 mg a day up to 20 mg per day).

Ebixa (NMDA, n-methyl-D-aspartate) is a "receptor antagonist." This amino acid derivate reacts as an agonist at the NMDA receptor sites. It creates an effect similar to the neurotransmitter glutamate, noted to be involved in transmitting nerve signals (important for learning and memory). Thus, changing the levels of glutamate can contribute to reducing symptoms observed in AD.

Before taking Ebixa, notify your physician if you have any medical conditions, including heart problems, uncontrolled hypertension (high blood pressure), a history of seizures or kidney disease; any medications, including prescriptions and nonprescriptions, that you are currently taking or have taken within the last fourteen days; if you have ever had an allergic reaction to any medication; if you have a urinary tract infection or kidney problems; if you have recently changed your diet substantially (e.g., from a diet including meat to a vegetarian diet); or if you smoke.

Cognex

Cognex (tacrine): This drug is not actively marketed by the manufacturer but is still available.

Cognex is another cholinesterase inhibitor designed to treat symptoms of AD. Cognex prevents the breakdown of acetylcholinesterase, thus increasing the amount of acetylcholine in the brain. This was the first AD drug approved by the FDA; however, it has limited use these days due to three main reasons: it must be taken four times daily, it has a number of unpleasant side effects (nausea, diarrhea), and it may cause serious liver damage.

Your physician should always be notified if you are on any other medications. All of these medications take as long as twelve weeks before benefit is observed; however, as with any medication, times can vary.

Finally, I have provided this list as a general guideline for individuals to understand what is generally known about these medications. The examples of quantities taken are just that—an example of common dosages. The reader should also be aware that new medications are in the development stage, and current medications are continuously followed to ensure the best possible outcomes. Thus, changes in recommended treatment programs may vary as the research unfolds.

9

WHAT IS MILD COGNITIVE IMPAIRMENT?

After reading this chapter, you should be able to answer the following questions:

If I have MCI, will I get AD?
What are the two subtypes of MCI?
What areas of my brain are affected?
How do I know if I have MCI?

Mild cognitive impairment (MCI) is a condition that can affect an individual's memory retrieval, visuospatial performance, and language and attention skills below the expected normal performance for that individual's given ability, but without significantly interfering with everyday functioning. Two subtypes of MCI have been identified: amnestic (predominately affecting memory) and nonamnestic (not significantly affecting memory).

MCI often becomes a concern as a result of self-realization, in that individuals begin to believe that their normal ability is somewhat impaired. These individuals normally have good insight and a good understanding of their abilities and are usually the first to say something does not seem right. They often report to primary-care centers with complaints that their performance is below what they expect of themselves. These are complaints related to one aspect of their life only (e.g., memory or language) and not two or more. Two or more areas of concern would move these individuals into a category involving a dementia diagnosis. Thus, the hallmark of MCI is that it is a deficit in one area of functioning and not several, unlike, for example, Alzheimer's disease, where two or more areas of concern would be needed for a diagnosis.

As noted above, there are currently two subtypes for this illness. Amnestic MCI refers to the fact that the individual is having a problem strictly relating to an aspect of memory, but no other deficits outside of this concern are noted. With nonamnestic MCI, concerns are related to a cognitive area not relying on memory, such as attention, language-finding ability, or visually guided movements. Remember, these concerns must be out of the ordinary and must be significantly impacting one's ability to perform at a normal, everyday level. This does not mean, for instance, that if you forgot where you placed your car keys twice last week, you must have a mild cognitive impairment. It is important to remember that it has to significantly affect your everyday functioning and, based on your "normal" functioning, seem very out of the ordinary, to the extent that you notice it impacting your life. An example might be forgetting where you placed your keys four times a week for the last few weeks, and noticing that they turn up in the freezer or microwave oven. If you never forgot your keys before and this is impacting your ability to perform everyday activities, then this could be a concern and you need to be evaluated for MCI or another illness. Please keep in mind that I have offered this example just as a guideline of a type of behavior that might fall into the realm of MCI or possible dementia.

We as humans personalize information in an effort to understand it and to make sense of it. Thus, when receiving a diagnosis of, for instance, MCI, we do not often ask what pathologically is going on in my brain. Usually what we want to know is how it's going to affect us (i.e., behaviorally). How am I going to function every day? What does the future hold? What can I do? And will this be noticeable to everyone around me? These are just some of the questions individuals often have when faced with a diagnosis. I will address these questions at the conclusion of this chapter, but first let's focus on the brain and understand pathologically what is occurring to give us some insight into what might be contributing to an MCI deficit.

PATHOLOGY OF MCI

This would be an extremely easy chapter to write if we could say that X causes Y. However, like most things in neuroscience, it is never that simple. I think one group of researchers said it best when they noted that "there is no silver bullet" at this time that fits the diverse pathologic, molecular, and cellular constellation of events that occur in the MCI brain.[1] There are a number of bad events happening as your brain and body age, and several of these events *may* impact your cognitive ability and lead to a cognitive impairment such as MCI or, even more drastically, a dementia-related illness. Which events specifically are responsible for causing an MCI deficit are not known for sure, and in reality it is more likely that it takes a number of events working together (synergistically) to cause the progression to cognitive impairment. In addition, how an individual's brain reacts to these "negative" events can be influenced, I believe, by what the individual has historically done and is currently doing to protect his or her health (brain and body). As researchers, we are not sure what triggers MCI, and it could be one or several things, leading to a cascade of issues creating cognitive disruption in one's brain. Individuals will not know what is occurring, for example, on a chemical level in their brains; they may, however, receive behavioral feedback though a reduction in certain abilities. In the case of MCI, this behavioral impact can be minimal and may be a warning sign of what *might* be on the horizon. In the following sections, I have highlighted a few of these events that could be underway. However, please remember these are examples of what could be occurring (and are by no means an exhaustive list). Again, each individual is exactly that—individual—and how the brain responds will be quite different from one person to the next.

Neurofibrillary Tangles

In Alzheimer's disease pathology, it is currently suggested, based on postmortem examinations of several individuals' brains who were afflicted with Alzheimer's disease and who displayed neurofibrillary tangles (NFT) throughout the progression of the illness, that the disease follows a certain staging process.[2] MCI individuals have selective areas affected by these tangles, and they are not as widespread as you would see in AD cases. Areas affected in MCI individuals are primarily in the hippocampus, an area noted for memory, and in the parietal areas, concerned with sensory perception, language, and sensorimotor integration (which can affect your visually guided movements).[3] This pathology of events (as it relates only to NFTs) fits well with behavioral explanations provided above and could be one of the primary issues in an MCI brain.

Amyloid

Beta-amyloid plaques, when seen widespread across the brain, are one of the primary links in our understanding of what is affecting neural transmission in Alzheimer's disease. In regard to MCI, these plaques are present, but until they move into the neurons the effects are minimal.[4] In fact, individuals with MCI and some with no identified deficits have shown significant amounts of beta-amyloid plaques in their brains in postmortem examinations, but without the cognitive impairments observed in, for example, an individual with Alzheimer's disease. Thus, the link between the pathology and behavior is not clear.[5] So trying to use beta-amyloid as a biological marker to distinguish a normal individual from an MCI individual does not appear to be a valid process.[6] However, what does appear to be important about these plaques is that once they move into specific areas of the brain, affecting neurons directly (neuritic plaques), and move deeper into the cortex, individuals are more likely to experience cognitive difficulties, and thus show behavioral deficits that could then be identified as MCI. The role of these amyloid plaques is to stop transmission between brain regions. However, dynamic brains have more than one route along which to send information between regions. Thus, for some individuals a greater amount plaque development (specifically, neuritic plaques) may need to be present to cause behavioral disruption. Without this behavioral change, it's highly unlikely individuals would be aware there was an issue or actually have themselves checked out for dementia-related concerns.

MCI, Plasticity, and Neurons

As has been noted in various places in this book, neurogenesis (or synaptogenesis) plays an important part in maintaining a healthy brain.

We all have the ability to create new neurons, and we all have the capacity for brain plasticity at any age. This ability, from a neuropathological standpoint, often becomes disrupted in conjunction with forms of neurodegenerative disease such as AD or MCI. In fact, research has shown that brain plasticity is affected in AD and MCI cases via reductions in proteins such as PSD95 and F-actin, both of which play an important role in stimulating neurogenesis.[7] Thus, slowing or interrupting neurogenesis can create impairments such as MCI, which I would suggest could be a result of a neurogenic imbalance (good brain processes affected by bad habits within one's brain)—but only to a certain extent, in that the effects of a full disease state are not significantly present. In addition, what might be more prominent in these cases is vascular issues (i.e., the blood vessels or blood flow affected). Many subtypes of dementia are now being linked to small or large blood vessel disruptions. These disruptions can set the stage for the development of MCI or a more serious dementia disease.[8] As researchers and clinicians move forward, this can and should be examined in each individual case.

Another issue recently examined in individuals with MCI is what's occurring in the receptor areas between neurons that want to talk to each other. Researchers have been trying to establish whether the neurons doing the talking (transmission) are having problems sending the message or the neurons listening (binding) are having trouble getting the message. There are of course many types of receptors and different types of chemicals (neurotransmitters) being transmitted between neurons. However, the one primarily of interest in both AD and MCI is acetylcholine (pronounced uh-seet-i-koh-leen). Acetylcholine tells the other neuron to get moving and send the signal; it needs to get the job done quickly because it has a short lifespan and is terminated quickly by acetylcholinesterase. In AD this has been studied fairly extensively, and many of the current medications used to combat symptoms of dementia are designed to increase available acetylcholine, which is an attempt to increase signals between neurons. In MCI, however, there has not been a significant amount of work done on these cases. Research has shown that if an MCI individual has a deficit in the binding site (message receiver site), they are most likely to progress to AD.[9] Why this is so is currently not known, but if this can be examined more closely to determine why it is happening in early-stage MCI, then it may provide some clues to how the process could be stopped or possibly reversed.

IDENTIFYING MCI

One of the major issues with identifying individuals with MCI is that they can often evolve into other disease states. This certainly does not mean that MCI is the link to other neurological diseases, but in many instances it has been identified as a precursor. Be aware that this is not always the case, and some individuals will maintain an MCI diagnosis for the duration of their life and thus never transition into a different disease state. However, arguments about this process vary widely.

Despite the information available, one of the primary questions individuals receiving an MCI diagnosis have is, If I have MCI, will I automatically progress to AD? Well, the quick answer is that not all MCI individuals will develop a dementia-related illness, but they are at an increased risk.[10] People recognize that cognitive impairment, including its symptoms, can be closely related to AD. Thus, there is great fear, and rightly so, among these individuals. They need and want to know what this means for them going forward. A clear understanding of what having MCI means varies. Below, I specifically outline some of the evidence of a connection between MCI and AD.

Researchers have shown that a combination of things can indicate if someone will progress from MCI to AD. One prominent example is biomarkers (biological evidence obtained, for example, through the collection of cerebrospinal fluid [CSF]). Results have shown that the risk of progression to AD was substantially increased in patients diagnosed with MCI who showed pathological concentrations of T-tau (genetic material that clogs the feeding routes of neurons) and Abeta42 (plaques affecting neuron signaling) at baseline. A combination of CSF T-tau and Abeta42 at baseline yielded a sensitivity of 95 percent and a specificity of 83 percent for the detection of incipient AD. Thus, the combination of this material, if observed in MCI, indicates a good chance that you will progress to AD.[11] Researchers determine if one has these specific genetic abnormalities via an examination of one's CSF, a bodily fluid located in the spinal cord and spaces around (subarachnoid space) and inside (ventricular system) the brain. This fluid essentially acts as protection for the brain. A lumbar puncture is performed to retrieve a sample of CSF. The procedure is often performed right in a physician's office. When you are diagnosed with MCI, biomarkers can provide insight into your susceptibility to AD, but as a patient you need to be wary of why you are being tested and what is being assessed. A lumbar puncture, because it is performed below the spinal cord in the L3/L4 area, where only nerve endings are located, has little risk of causing paralysis. This danger has been greatly exaggerated based on the location of CSF fluid. However, the danger in many clinical settings is very low. General practicing physicians will most likely not take a CSF sample, and if they did, they most likely would not have a lab that has the expertise to evaluate the sample to determine risk levels and the aforementioned genetic markers. It is important, however, to be aware of these biomarkers, and that they can help an individual prepare and understand what is to come. Finally, I should also note that a lumbar puncture is a very painful procedure and can include side effects such as severe headache and stiffness, so understanding all your options and your end goal is important before proceeding.

There are, of course, other ways researchers try to evaluate the likelihood of an individual transitioning from MCI to AD. One of the best noninvasive ways to do this is through neuroimaging markers. Researchers measure cortical thickness in certain brain locations to determine the likelihood that one will continue to progress to full-blown AD. This type of measurement and others are normally used in conjunction with behavioral measures in an effort to identify relationships between what can be seen in the brain and what this means behaviorally. One study examined MRI imaging to determine cortical thickness in patients and then determined how they were performing to understand the likelihood that certain individuals would progress to AD. Interestingly, they suggest that if there is a reduction in cortical thickness in one's right inferior temporal lobe and a poor behavioral score (less than 15.67) on the Alzheimer's Disease Assessment Scale (ADAS13), then this is a good indication that an individual will convert to AD. In fact, they indicated rates on average of 92.7 percent resulting in a conversion to AD with this level of behavioral score, and an 88.8 percent rate of conversion to AD if one's cortical thickness was significantly reduced (smaller than 2.56 mm^3).[12] As with CSF, evaluating one's cortical thickness is still a difficult prospect, especially if your primary-care physician does not have access to the necessary MRI equipment or the expertise to measure cortical thickness properly. As mentioned above, a true diagnosis of possible or probable AD will include a neuroimaging examination, at which point one could ascertain cortical thickness in certain brain regions. However, this type of evaluation is not often undertaken in MCI cases, and with health-care resources already at a significant strain, care of this nature may be difficult to get or not be very timely if it does occur.

MCI AND THE EVERYDAY

Finally, to conclude this chapter, I would like to address the questions I posed earlier: How am I going to function every day? What does the future hold? What can I do? And will this be noticeable to everyone around me? These are just some of the questions individuals often have when faced with a diagnosis of MCI. Well, first of all, the good news about MCI is that it is a *mild* impairment, and thus there is generally not a significant impact on one's life, as would be the case with a dementia diagnosis. The general complaint individuals have about MCI is that they are the ones who are aware that they are not functioning at a normal level. Therefore, most likely the individuals around them will not be aware of any issues unless the individual points it out. As for functioning every day, because MCI individuals are generally aware of their deficits, they can devise strategies to compensate when needed. For example, if they were used to remembering implicitly when they had an appointment, they could alter this behavior by using an external device such as a digital scheduling system to remind them of their appointments. If remembering general information such as a friend's address seems difficult, then they might compensate by carrying a standard information sheet for certain important information.

As for one's future, that becomes a difficult question. Could someone continue with MCI for a significant amount of time? Certainly. Could he or she transition to a dementia-related illness? The answer is also yes. As for what one can do, one can get active, both cognitively and physically, as well as watch what one eats and have an understanding of the benefits of certain activities and foods. I have within this book provided some suggestions around physical and cognitive exercise that are beneficial for everyone to engage in, especially as they age, to potentially avoid conditions such as MCI, but if you have been given a diagnosis, I would start engaging in all that I have suggested as soon as possible, simply because I foresee nothing but great benefits. And the sooner one gets going, the better chance the brain will have. Please note that although I have highlighted ways to achieving a healthy brain in this book, I am simply providing examples of ways to get there, but there is always more than one path. If you have a plan and it works well for you, then go with it. Make sure you understand the ins and outs of your plan and the schedule you have devised. Remember that you are the person who will know best how things are working for you.

10

HOW DO I KNOW IF MY BRAIN IS AGING NORMALLY?

After reading this chapter, you should be able to answer the following questions:

Does my intelligence alter as I age?

In which decade of my life might I expect a change in my cognitive ability?

Is there an age limit at which having a healthy brain is no longer possible?

Will age-related reduction in brain volume result in a cognitive decline?

AGING CONCERNS

Aging individuals are often concerned if they are aging at a rate that seems relatively comparable to their peers. However, depending on the person and their past experiences, the focus of successful aging can, and will be, quite different. For example, individuals are interested in understanding various issues, such as: Am I as fast a runner/walker as other people my age? Is my golf score the same as others my age? I wonder how my *Jeopardy* performance was this week; am I still quicker and better at answering questions than others my age? The point is that individuals use what they know to measure change, which for many is based on a personal history of stable performance, providing them with a good understanding of what their performance should normally be. A majority of us use our normal performance as a benchmark to identify if things are different from normal. Of course, this will alter somewhat as we age, but for the most part individuals are attuned to how they are likely to perform on any given task. In fact, when explaining concerns to anyone, including a family physician, why you believe something is substantially different is often accompanied with a report. For example, "Well, I used to remember all the names of the seven dwarfs alphabetically, but now I have real trouble remembering their names at all." Changes like this lead people to wonder, Am I the same person, or have I lost some ability? Is this normal? This in turn results in several other questions: Is this temporary? Will I get worse? How concerned should I be? These are important concerns all aging individuals share. The real problem for many is distinguishing the normal from the abnormal. I will discuss various ways this can be achieved throughout this chapter.

To begin, I want to review the concept of variations in cognitive performance and what is currently viewed as normal cognitive ability as one ages. Then I will look at the general structural changes observed in the brain as one ages, including how these structural changes might affect one's performance, and what we can, and should do, to offset this process.

VARYING COGNITIVE ABILITY

Like the majority of things in our world, there is inherent variability in aging, meaning in this case that all individuals are not the same. As individuals age, they will change at varying rates. This includes, of course, one's cognitive ability. Therefore, it cannot be assumed that if you are old, you have this kind or that kind of cognitive deficit by default. Individuals are just that, individual, and strengths and weakness you possessed when you were younger are most likely similar to the ones you are more aware of as you age. Is it a factor of age that makes these more prevalent, or is it a lifetime of experience recognizing what you are good at and what you are not good at that makes your deficits more apparent? It may be that many aging individuals are quite aware of the deficits they have, and as such they do not even attempt tasks they know they are not good at. One might wonder why. Well, it could be that there is no joy in doing something you do not want to do, or they have come to terms with their poor performance (in whatever task it could be for that person) and they neither have the time nor the will to challenge themselves anymore, especially when it can be completed by someone else or a machine (e.g., a calculator for simple math). For the most part, aging individuals are not in school anymore, and no one is checking their homework, so if they are not being challenged, then they will have no reason or desire to complete tasks they know are not enjoyable. Could these be reasons that individuals exhibit certain deficits? Possibly. But this has not been clearly demonstrated to date. Thus, I have included this preamble just as food for thought as I present some of the research involved in varying cognitive ability as we age below.

Before examining some of the current research being conducted, I would like to point out that cognitive ability, or intelligence as used by some researchers, refers to different modalities, and these modalities (e.g., perception, memory, judgment, spatial manipulation) are often used together either to make composite scores that represent one's ability in a specific cognitive domain (e.g., organization ability) or to provide an assessment of overall performance. These types of evaluations are very common and provide researchers with the ability to look at distinctions in certain cognitive areas or in overall ability. Research has suggested that cognitive performance changes as one ages.[1] Intelligence can be measured through two fundamental processes: fluid and crystallized. Fluid intelligence refers to an individual's ability to solve novel problems, to think logically, identifying patterns in mental speed tasks. Crystallized intelligence refers to one's general knowledge store, vocabulary, and word knowledge and is often noted to be rooted in one's educational and vocational experiences. These distinctions are important because research has shown that crystallized intelligence remains relatively stable throughout the majority of adult life (twenty-five to seventy years old). Fluid intelligence results, however, are quite different. For example, in completing a task such as coding speed (pattern identification), significant differences can be observed between younger and older participants. How much cognitive decline can one expect as one ages? Well, these researchers suggest that at an overall group level there is a fifteen to thirty IQ point decline, particularly in fluid intelligence, from one's twenties to seventies. After seventy, the decline in fluid abilities is not as dramatic and may move on average 7.5 points for each decade.[2]

One of the main difficulties in research of this kind is controlling for environmental influences. Though researchers can examine variations within the population and control for these factors, one of hardest things to control for is environment; because experiences are so varied, it is very difficult to ensure participants share similar environmental experiences. With this in mind, further controlled evaluations have been undertaken to address these concerns, with the priority of understanding how cognitive changes affect individuals in their later years.

Controlling for environmental circumstances is clearly difficult; however, a creative way this issue has been addressed is by using participants from institutions (e.g., religious organizations). One such study used participants from religious orders.[3] Researchers examined over a six-year period changes in the cognitive abilities of 694 catholic clergy, which included nuns, priests, and brothers. Overall results showed a decline in cognitive ability as individuals moved from their sixties to seventies (averaging a 0.03 unit of decline) and from their seventies to eighties (averaging a 0.011 unit of decline). However, as you can see, the average rate of cognitive decline in this study was relativity small. Researchers suggested that this could be due to exclusion of individuals experiencing dementia-related disturbance at baseline (the start of the study). Individuals who experienced a decline in one cognitive area were more likely to experience a decline in another. This result led researchers to conclude that cognitive decline is more likely a global factor and not very selective. Interestingly, these researchers also noted that individual variability in rates of change included improvement, similar performance, and gradual and sharp decline. Thus, basically every type of change that could be observed was observed on an individual level. An important limitation of this research (as pointed out by the authors) was that these individuals were a selective group. Thus, it may prove difficult to generalize the results to the population at large. Though this group was highly selective, the findings are still very interesting, in that small declines were noted and the majority of individuals continued to perform at a fairly decent cognitive level. I think additional evidence related to daily activities, including diet, exercise level, and engagement in cognitive activities for all involved, would provide greater insight into what influenced performance change.

Researchers have been interested in understanding dynamitic changes that occur in cognitive ability and their subsequent brain functions. One study in particular examined changes in cognitive performance and brain function in a participant sample of individuals with an average age of sixty-eight. Results showed that over the eight-year period, there was no overall change in cognitive ability; however, examination using PET imaging showed that when completing recognition memory tasks increases in brain response were observable in both the temporal and parietal regions. This was in contrast to the parahippocampal, temporal, and frontal regions, where reduced activation was noted.[4]

Other researchers have reported, in a review article on successful aging, that increased brain activation is generally linked to better cognitive performance. As well, a positive relationship in ability was normally seen in individuals with increased responsiveness in the frontal lobe. As for the parietal and temporal areas, research suggests a more mixed result, but with several studies indicating the presence of a positive relationship.[5] One suggestion would be that activation within the frontal cortex increases to handle deficits within other brain areas. However, there would have to be a deficit occurring in the first place to trigger this increase in activation and the subsequent compensatory action. Thus, altered activation might suggest an impending cognitive concern. Therefore, a more stable pattern of brain activity with limited fluctuations either positive or negative may in fact be a sign of healthy cognitive aging.

The above research provides a good account of the types of cognitive changes healthy individuals may face as they advance in age. But one question you might still have is, what about the very old, individuals around one hundred years old? (You might be there, or want to be there someday.) Though rather rare a few decades back, it is becoming relatively more common for individuals to reach this advanced age. One important question aging individuals are interested in knowing is, Am I guaranteed to have a cognitive deficit when I reach the age of ninety-five or one hundred? This question is becoming more and more relevant as the majority of industrialized nations' average life expectancy rates continue to rise. Not surprisingly, researchers have begun to examine cognitive performance in the very old or, the term I prefer, the very mature.

As an aging individual, should one expect to automatically have a cognitive impairment after reaching the age of one hundred? The good news is no. But if you are not guaranteed to have a cognitive deficit at that age, what are the chances that I will have a cognitive deficit at one hundred? Numerous researchers in several countries around the world have suggested that anywhere between 40 to 62 percent of individuals ninety-five or older will demonstrate some form of moderate to severe cognitive impairment.[6] Though this is not great news for this group, there is some good news: the same researchers also showed that between 20 and 25 percent of centenarians experienced no cognitive deficits whatsoever. The remaining individuals were said to be at a borderline stage. Longitudinal research of centenarians demonstrates that at an eighteen-month follow-up, with the exception of a few cases, this group had not experienced any significant decline.[7] These results, the first of their kind, demonstrate that cognitive stability could be observed even in this "very mature," and most notably, about a quarter of them were still functioning at a normal cognitive level. Further examination of this data noted that at the first testing session, those still living had cognitive scores similar to those who died before the next session, indicating that cognitive decline is relatively stable in this group and does not provide insight into predicting mortality among centenarians. This result is interesting because in younger age groups (e.g., sixty-five to eighty years old) cognitive decline has been associated with impending death, to the extent that it has even been suggested that accelerated cognitive decline is for this age group an indicator of rapidly approaching death.[8] Finally, it is important to note that these effects were observed in normally aging individuals (healthy adults). Individuals who already had a dementia-related illness were not influencing the results. Though this might seem to be a worrisome point, I certainly believe that one has the ability to be in that 25 percent of cognitively healthy centenarians, and the information provided in this book will point you in the right direction.

AGING BRAIN STRUCTURE

One of the most difficult tasks for researchers is identifying the link between structural brain changes and the resulting effect on an individual's cognitive performance. As previously stated, regional brain areas do not work in isolation from one another but operate through a multitude of neural connections. That being said, change often occurs or begins in specific brain regions. Because certain regions are highly involved in generating specific responses, many researchers examine task-driven brain areas. Examining structural changes in the brain related to deterioration (shrinkage) as a result of the normal aging process is one way to help understand the performance difficulties aging individuals might face.

One of the common cognitive complaints reported by researchers is that aging individuals often indicate that their memory is "not what it used to be." The majority of healthy aging individuals will follow up this statement with something like, "But, all and all, it's not that bad. I just forget some little things here and there, like remembering to pick up milk when I am at the store." Because memory complaints are more readily recognizable and noticeable to aging individuals, they have historically been the focus of research and, as such, the focus on structural brain research as it relates to cognitive performance.

Aging individuals also often report that they perseverate (get caught up) in performing certain tasks. Perseveration is often observed to increase with age and has been linked to normal age-related structural shrinkage of the prefrontal cortex.[9] Thus, declining ability to task switch (move from one task to another), based on current research, is a factor in general aging and not related to the presence or development of a specific disease. It is important to note that the sample group in this study had an average age of forty-four (plus or minus sixteen years), as well as having an average of sixteen years of education (plus or minus two). This is interesting because it suggests that quite earlier on our brains begin to change structurally, which can subsequently result in altered cognitive processing. Researchers also demonstrated that cortical regions primarily responsible for supporting working memory (specifically, the visual cortex and fusiform gyrus, a region spanning both the temporal and occipital lobes) are also susceptible to cortical shrinkage as we age.[10] Working-memory tasks can be verbal or nonverbal; however, the result of cortical shrinkage in this study primarily affected nonverbal performance. Nonverbal working-memory tasks involve such things as organizing and grouping long lists of items in your mind, or tasks such as using object pieces to assemble structures (e.g., puzzles). This study also reported as a result of shrinkage of the visual cortex and fusiform gyrus additional functionality/cognitive deficits. For example, explicit memory procedures. These are tasks such as associating new names to new items (not previously presented, these are usually made-up items) or recalling the elements of a short narrative story and repeating as many details as possible back to the researcher. Tasks of this nature, not surprisingly since these are some of the first kinds of memory complaints reported, are thought to be linked to cortical brain shrinkage.[11] Therefore, subtle decreases in one's performance might be linked to internal physiological aspects of aging. Though this is compelling evidence, it is important to note that differences observed may be so subtle that many of us would not be aware of them without participating in ongoing testing. Though cortical shrinkage may occur for many healthy aging individuals, the process is often limited, and functional disruptions can often go unnoticed. This can be for the simple reason that the healthy aging brain has efficient neural processing, and many different avenues to send and receive information, a factor attributed to healthy brains and often a result of "brain experience." In addition, it should also be pointed out that, as one ages, one's physical abilities can also be affected, including many sensory modalities such as hearing and vision, which may also contribute to the reduced performance rates observed in this research. Thus, research controlling for these factors and examining specific processes involved in cognitive performance as one ages is of great interest. Examining individual variations that can occur in healthy individuals as a result of the normal aging process is very important to us all, and will be the primary focus for the rest of this chapter.

HOW DO I STOP MY BRAIN FROM SHRINKING?

One very important question to be addressed is, If my brain is shrinking simply because I am aging, is there a way to build it back up? Yes! There are ways to maintain your brain's health even as one ages. Physiologists have shown that your body begins to break down as you age. One example of what occurs as you age is losing a significant amount of muscle mass, which is directly linked to our bodies' "standard" aging process. However, there are ways to offset this breakdown. For instance, how much muscle mass you lose can be reduced significantly by regularly engaging in weight training activities.[12] Though your brain is the most complex organ known to man, if you exercise it, like the rest of your muscles, you can offset reductions. Though the exercise process is somewhat different, the concept of regular attention is the same. Similar to making time to go to the gym, lift weights, and get on the treadmill (see chapter 11 for example activities), which helps ensure consistent health, we also need to exercise our brain. If there was such a thing as a "Brain Gym," I would recommend joining it as much as, if not more than, a regular gym.

You might ask yourself, Can a little training really affect my brain structure and cortical composition? First, it is important to state as noted earlier, there is inherent variability, and some individuals may require more training than others to reach similar levels as their peers. Regardless, current evidence indicates that adults on an individual level have the ability to change their cortical structure and generate new brain growth. In fact, researchers from the University of Hong Kong demonstrated that having adults engage in a simple learning task (similar to one used with children, with one simple twist), where a color card is presented and participants are required to state the color's name, resulted in neural growth. Researches altered the task by providing made-up names for each of the colors presented and then having participants learn these new names to be tested on later. The university student participants were given MRI scans before the three days of training, which consisted of five sessions totalling only two hours. Remarkably, the MRI scans conducted after training showed that all nineteen participants formed new gray matter in their left hemispheres (mainly visual cortex) within this very short period.[13] What is also remarkable about these findings is that the task did not require a significant amount of effort or time, suggesting that the important task component was the novelty of word names linked to known colors. With the introduction of new names for standard colors, new associations were required, which facilitated the need to relearn and remap associations, which in turn was thought to stimulate brain growth. It is also important to note that these participants were not children, proving that real neural growth can still be observed in adult populations.

This study provides one example of how structural changes can be positively altered with cognitive interventions. How about physical interventions? I do not mean opening up the skull and stretching your brain, though that is an interesting thought. Rather, does physical exercise actually produce change in the size of certain brain structures? As it so happens, researchers have shown that brain structure can be altered through such exercise. In this research, 120 adults (with a mean age of sixty-six years old) participated in either an aerobic exercise (consisting of walking for forty minutes, three days a week) or a stretching program. What they found after following the participants for one year was that individuals in the aerobic exercise group had increased the structural volume of their hippocampus (the main structure involved in memory) by 2 percent. Researchers indicated that this should result in offsetting deterioration of this region associated with general aging by about one to two years. This result was opposed to the stretching group, who had a 1.4 percent decline in the same brain region, suggesting that you can turn the clock back and maintain or even regain lost brain volume. Consequently, this study also demonstrated improved memory function in the aerobic group, suggesting that brain volume may be directly linked to cognitive performance.[14]

Animal models provide additional support to the theory that the brain can grow and change even in the face of deficits occurring at critical periods. Critical periods generally occur during development, when there is extensive neural growth. A basic example is individuals with hearing deficits, who in early life can have language difficulties (e.g., pronunciation, reading, etc.). These sensory deficits can substantially affect cognitive development. Historically, the belief has been that missing critical periods can have a lifelong impact. More recently, we have seen that with extensive training, many of these deficits can be overcome. For example, researchers have shown that rats reared in environments designed to disrupt the animal's ability to process different types of sound, allowing for the development of an abnormal brain structure, can overcome this difficulty. Researchers were able to change this developmental deficit with extensive training, which successfully restored cortical and behavioral function in animals that missed a critical development period. These researchers were also able to restore function in both juveniles and adults.[15] This type of evidence lends further support to the idea that even in the face of advancing age or the loss of skill development at critical periods, the capacity to alter actual brain structure and grow new neurons in support of strengthening or building cortical connections is a reality and not science fiction.

If we are all aging, and a reduction in our brain structure or volume is inevitable, some people might think they are doomed and that, if they do nothing, their cognitive skills will be significantly impacted. This is not exactly true. Many of us know individuals who have not lost much cognitive ability at all and others who have lost a lot. People often ask, Is bigger better? Is there a direct link to age-related brain volume decline and poor cognitive ability? The answer to these questions is that we really do not know. Results to date have been conflicting, and researchers have not demonstrated consistently that age-related reduction in brain volume will result in cognitive decline. What is known is that age-related volume decline will occur but is often confined to specific brain regions, leaving the various results open to interpretation.[16] When positive relationships are observed between increased brain structure/volume and increased cognitive ability, the conclusion is bigger is better. However, because only certain structures will be bigger, researchers speculate that this one area helps compensate for other regions experiencing difficulty.[17] Conversely, when a negative relationship is observed, in that poor cognitive performance is associated with increased brain volume, the conclusion is that poor neural pruning has occurred.[18] But during brain development, many of these neural connections are not being used properly. A more plausible reason for an observed negative relationship between brain volume and performance ability is that these older, healthy individuals have high "cognitive reserves," which suggests that their brains work more efficiently and effectively using only a limited and minimal amount of cortical resources. You may wonder why that is, and the simple answer is because they can. If you can do more with less, that is a successful strategy in managing resources.[19] With age comes experience, and your brain becomes quite adept at performing a variety of tasks, making some tasks more cognitively taxing than others. Utilizing these resources becomes an everyday skill for many individuals and, subsequently, for their brains.

Many researchers believe that chronological age has its limitations. For instance, it might tell us nothing intuitively about an individual's cognitive or physical ability. However, understanding an individual's biological age can provide a better understanding of where an individual exists on life's continuum.[20] This is a valuable point for a couple of reasons. First, individuals often report feeling healthy and can display good cognitive abilities but might question this ability because all their life they have been told, when you reach a certain age, you are not going to be able to do this or that. The second point I believe affects a number of younger individuals, but in the opposite way. They might believe that because they are only a certain age, they should not be experiencing any difficulties and, as such, can ignore warning signs telling them their lifestyle is hurting their health. Researchers have been trying to examine cognitive age by linking this to an individual's biological age. Key ways this has been achieved is through the examination of health biomarkers such as muscle strength (diminished grip), cardiovascular health (increased systolic accompanied with lower diastolic pressure), and body composition (declining body mass). These measures have been correlated to the presence of a cognitive impairment. Specifically, the strongest link was to individuals' deficits in semantic memory.[21] Thus, one's level of health on these domains can be linked to mental ability. This type of research is still in its early stages, and the goal moving forward is to look specifically at alternations (variants) in genetic makeup to determine how the presence of, for example, inflammation, homocysteine concentrations, or increased levels of oxidative stress can affect one's cognitive ability long term.[22] In time, individuals, as part of their health workup, will have the option to have their genome sequenced, which can give individuals insight into illnesses they may be susceptible to as they age. In the future, this sequencing might also have the ability to test for susceptibility to cognitive impairment. I should note that having your whole genome sequence is currently available through private firms, and the cost can range from fifteen to forty thousand dollars. The real issue is the interpretation of the results, which are generally described to the individual as a predisposition. Thus you can have a predisposition or a susceptibility that is higher than average. For example, you could be at an increased risk for cardiovascular disease. This does not mean you will certainly get this illness, but the hope of researchers is that it will provide evidence and a warning sign that, if symptoms appear, you should seek treatment as soon as possible. This is certainly the positive side to the process, and it will help individuals remain vigilant of an illness that may develop.

I have provided a number of examples throughout of how one's brain may be affected by age. These are by no means hard-and-fast rules. Everyone starts from a different base, and when judging performance, there is a need to be reflective on how you have performed historically. One example in this chapter was aging individuals who observed difficulty in maintaining their nonverbal ability. It was noted that these types of procedures are observed to be deficient in individuals of advanced age. But the nonverbal ability of, for example, using object pieces for the purpose of putting something back together is a reoccurring and ongoing deficit someone might possess. An individual, therefore, might never perform well on such tasks, and to use this as a measure of how successfully he or she is aging would not be sufficient or appropriate. Assessing one's ability in relation to age-related peers can be difficult, and sometimes the best marker is your own performance. Keep in mind that age and education benchmarks can be most useful in providing a holistic understanding of your abilities and provide insight as you age.

Section III

Healthy Living as We Age

11

EXERCISE AND DIET

After reading this chapter, you should be able to answer the following questions:

Is there really such a thing as brain food?

Do vitamins C, A, D, and E actually contain antiaging properties?

Can vitamins C, A, D, and E alter the course of cognitive impairments?

Can resveratrol promote brain health and affect the process of certain neurodegenerative diseases?

Is a calorie-restrictive diet one way to ensure a healthy brain?

Is exercise an effective way to fight and prevent cognitive impairments, and, if so, how much is enough?

The overall message the general public receives is that if one eats well and exercises, one should be able to maintain good physical health, good mobility, and intact mental faculties. In this chapter, I will discuss specific neuroprotective effects in relation to diet and exercise and try to unravel why we need to be wary of what we ingest, why we need to get up and get moving, and why we need to watch what we eat.

VITAMINS

Every so often, journalists will discover a medical study that can be transformed into a nightly news report or feature article. The focus of these reports is usually on some new type of therapy, a new "miracle drug," or how what we eat and certain vitamins we consume can affect our overall health. Globally, the human population is aging, to the extent that people over sixty-five will outnumber children under five most likely for the rest of human history.[1] As such, one of the areas of focus when it comes to aging well is identifying supplements that can positively affect the aging process, especially cell oxidation. *Oxidation* is a term often used when we talk about rust on a car; however, humans essentially also experience this process, though somewhat differently of course. Finding ways to fight this aging process is of great personal and commercial interest to the global community.

Oxidation occurs on a cellular level and is caused by a chemical reaction that stimulates the production of free radicals (unpaired electrons that can cause cellular damage). Free radicals within a cell basically cause damage or cell death. Thus, much research has examined how to stop this chemical reaction through the recruitment of antioxidants. Antioxidants do as they describe: they stop oxidation. Thus, foods rich in certain antioxidants are marketed as a way to maintain health and fight the aging process—hence so-called antiaging foods and vitamins. Historically, foods rich in vitamins C and E (noted to stimulate antioxidant enzymes) are often promoted as excellent and safe ways to reduce oxidative stress and increase cell health, thereby affecting one's overall health in a positive way.

Researchers have therefore been very interested in understanding the role of vitamins C, A, D, and particularly vitamin E in effecting change in "at risk populations," such as individuals with a neurodegenerative condition like Alzheimer's disease (AD) or mild cognitive impairment (MCI).

One might say that vitamin C was partly responsible for building the British Empire. This is because the British, among other nations, were exploring the world by sea, and one of the greatest obstacles they faced was maintaining the health of their sailors. The British discovered that eating fresh citrus fruit would help their sailors avoid scurvy, and with this discovery came the first controlled experiment of vitamin C. A Royal Navy surgeon, James Lind, confirmed that sailors given daily fresh citrus fruit remained healthy compared to another group of sailors who received their usual diet.[2] Since that time, it has become common knowledge that individuals should consume fresh fruit to ensure intake of vitamin C. Vitamin C (aka L-ascorbic acid) is a water-soluble vitamin important in healthy metabolic functioning. Because of its prominence, it is often consumed in large amounts, particularly in Western societies. A Canadian study showed that on average males ingest 133 mg per day and females 120 mg per day.[3] The recommended daily dose of vitamin C varies, but amounts close to 90 mg a day for males and 75 mg for females, give or take 10 mg, will be effective; for the elderly, it is recommend they maintain levels at the high end of this scale.[4] To ensure good levels, one should know that three-quarters of a cup of orange juice contains about 60 mg of vitamin C, so it is not difficult to maintain proper levels.

Vitamin C has also gained notoriety in positively affecting heart health (it helps produce collagen needed in the vascular system) and is also used by individuals with a family history of cancer, though definite links to effectiveness are still difficult to ascertain.[5] Clinical researchers have shown that vitamin C can contribute to a decreased risk of cardio-vascular disease and stroke by reducing systolic blood pressure.[6] As I will discuss later, though we know that our vascular system is essential in brain health, what we really want to know here is if vitamin C can help your brain. It is difficult to know for sure because, of all the organs in the body, the brain is the least likely to lose vitamin C derivatives (e.g., ascorbate). What this indicates is that vitamin C is essential in brain functioning. In addition, ascorbate is thought to be a neuromodulator for glutamatergic, dopaminergic, cholinergic, and GABAergic transmissions.[7] Finally, it is important to point out that neurodegenerative diseases often involve high levels of oxidative stress, and ascorbate is thought to help reduce free radicals and thus may be helpful in combating aging in general.[8]

Vitamin A affects a variety of functions throughout the body (e.g., vision, immune function, skin and cellular health, and antioxidant activity). Vitamin A deficiency affects vision development to the extent that approximately 250,000 to 500,000 children in regions such as southeast Asia and Africa become blind as a result.[9] Secondary problems associated with vitamin A deficiencies are linked to a reduction in one's immune system. In fact, studies in developing countries have shown that vitamin A deficiencies can be linked to significant increases in mortality rates for individuals afflicted with malaria.[10] Thus, its connection to health is well established.

Vitamin A is a fat-soluble vitamin. Therefore, removing extraneous amounts is more difficult than with vitamins C and B, which are water soluble. This means that individuals need to be wary of high doses that can create toxic levels. Currently, it is believed that doses exceeding 3,000 µg per day are not recommended for either sex. Suggested intake for females is 700 µg per day, and for males 900 µg per day.[11] It has also been suggested that individuals in developed nations may be ingesting more than the recommend daily amounts. Ingesting beyond the recommended amount has been linked to hip fractures and osteoporosis.[12]

So, can it help the brain? The general consensus to this answer is that there is no answer. Vitamin A's effectiveness in altering the course of cognitive impairment is not well defined, and as such no conclusions can be drawn.[13] So what we know about this vitamin in regard to maintenance of brain health is rather little. I believe that in the course of understanding the entire process of this vitamin, further insights will be explored and more answers will come.

Another vitamin that has been receiving a lot of attention as of late is D. Vitamin D has been noted to have a beneficial role in muscle function, cardiovascular health, diabetes, and cancer prevention.[14] Again, the links are not 100 percent. Additional evidence has suggested that vitamin D can be effective in cases where vascular factors (such as partially blocked arteries) are causing a cognitive impairment,[15] or as a protective agent against risk factors associated with cognitive dysfunction.[16] However, as has been the case with the other vitamins, a definite conclusion has not been reached. A systematic review of several studies evaluating the effectiveness of vitamin D, including its ability to maintain a therapeutic and consistent presence in the body, showed mixed results. For example, three studies displayed positive benefits, while eleven other studies showed nonsignificant relationships.[17] Though the verdict on vitamin D is still out, one should remain vigilant of new research outlining proper doses to consume and the achievable benefits to be gained through the use of this vitamin. It is my belief that it may have a number of benefits not fully understood to date.

Vitamin E is a fat-soluble antioxidant. Functions have been observed in relation to the regulation of enzyme activities involved with smooth muscle growth, gene expression, and connective tissue growth (meaning it is good for repairing wounds and tissue).[18] Most prominently, vitamin E is noted as an antioxidant for neural tissue. Research has shown that when one-year-old rats are stressed (injected with oxygen-derived free radicals), the organ affected first is the brain.[19] Thus, insufficient amounts of vitamin E can affect neuron growth, membrane formation, and cellular trafficking.[20] With this and other evidence in mind, researchers logically assume large amounts of vitamin E may be beneficial to the brain, especially for individuals in an at-risk group, such as those experiencing a cognitive impairment.

Thus, in the last decade or so, vitamin E has been described as an agent of change, and for several years it was, and often still is, prescribed as a way to augment medicative therapy for individuals experiencing a cognitive impairment. Vitamin E therefore became the standard recommended vitamin for many individuals receiving a diagnosis of cognitive impairment, particularly those with dementia. But what does the research tell us about vitamin E? The role of vitamin E as an effective antioxidant and in maintaining a healthy brain has not been substantiated to date. Vitamin E and vitamin C, as noted above, have important antioxidant properties, but their ability to produce effective change in individuals with dementia or as a neuroprotective strategy for those experiencing mild cognitive impairment has not been conclusively demonstrated.[21] A three-year follow-up study examining the effects of vitamin E on the onset of AD in subjects who already had a mild cognitive impairment showed no significant effects.[22] As well, long-term high doses of vitamin E (400 IU per day) increased mortality compared to low-dose trials.[23] Thus, as a standard of care for the treatment of AD, vitamin E is not as widely prescribed as it once was. In addition, greater care is now taken before recommending high doses of any vitamins, but especially vitamin E.

Finally, caution and common sense should be used when engaging in significantly high doses of specific vitamins. Their effects can be variable, and in some cases quite powerful, and therefore need to be approached with a certain amount of skepticism, especially given the research on vitamin E. People are often looking for an answer or a course of action, particularly when it comes to ingesting the appropriate type of vitamins, including knowing the proper dosages, proper combinations, and the best times of day to take them. As I have shown, there are no hard-and-fast answers, but that certainly does not mean that one should neglect vitamins either. To gain the full benefit of taking vitamins, you should ingest them before meals and not after, as it helps increase the absorption levels of other nutrients in your food. Vitamins have their role and can be effective for certain individuals more than others. For example, those who already eat a vitamin-rich diet may not benefit from extensive vitamin use; however, individuals with a diet that is vitamin deficient could experience good results. Finally, individuals who consume vitamins often engage in healthy behaviors to begin with, and thus at a population level it is difficult to understand their rate of effectiveness. What can be drawn from this is that healthy behaviors (e.g., regular exercise) and the use of vitamins (consumed through vitamin-rich foods) provide the advantage of a healthy life.

RESVERATROL

Resveratrol is another common subject of antiaging conversations. Resveratrol is a polyphenolic phytocompound of the stilbene family. So, basically, this is a chemical compound found in certain plants, and its role is to fight bacteria. However, when foods rich in resveratrol are consumed by humans, it has antioxidant benefits. Study of resveratrol came about when it was noticed that the French, whose diet is higher in fat (e.g., cheeses, pastries) than many other countries, still experienced a relatively low rate of cardiovascular disease.[24] This of course upset a number of other nations because it did not seem fair that the French were living with consequence-free diets, and in the interest of science, others were curious about what was happening. Researchers noticed that the French consumed a significant amount of wine, more than any other nation in fact, and especially red wine, and an initial link was established. Upon further investigation, it was found that red wine possessed an anticoagulate property, known as resveratrol. Therefore, although the French diet was terribly high in fat, it was being offset by the consumption of red wine.[25] Since this initial discovery, a number of additional foods have been identified as being high in resveratrol content, including red grapes, blueberries, cranberries, peanuts, Japanese knotweed, and dark chocolate (cocoa), just to name a few.[26] In addition, researchers have discovered that not only can one reap anticoagulate effects from resveratrol, but this compound may have neuroprotective properties.

Now before you grab your car keys and head to the store for some red wine and dark chocolate, you need to know a few things about resveratrol. One is that resveratrol metabolizes particularly fast, so fast that in a 25 mg oral dose less than 5 ng/ml (nanograms per milliliter) is measurable in your blood. What this means is that you would have to consume over four liters of red wine to reach a therapeutic level in a single dose.[27] However, resveratrol levels can have neuroprotective effects in derived concentrations ranging from 10 to 100 µM (100 µM is .00394 inches).[28] Researchers are still working on increasing its bioavailability (level it gets to in your body) to ensure that beneficial effects can be reached each time you take a dose.

However, what I am sure you really want to know is if resveratrol can help your brain. Well, the short answer is, yes, it appears that it can. Research has shown that resveratrol contains neuroprotective properties and is linked to longevity. One of the most interesting factors of resveratrol is that it has been shown to alter the course of AD. One of the primary genetic factors in AD is the production of beta-amyloid, which is the precursor to developing plaques and tangles in your brain (see chapter 6). Recent evidence has shown that beta-amyloid production is reduced when resveratrol is present.[29] The hope is that the progression of AD could be slowed significantly or stopped by refining the interactive process of certain chemical compounds (e.g., sirtuins) involved in promoting healthy cells. Currently, resveratrol is linked to the promotion of these healthy chemical compounds and continues to be examined, particularly in relation to neurodegenerative diseases. In fact, researchers have shown that production of healthy chemical compounds stemming from ingestion of resveratrol affects disease progression in other neurodegenerative conditions such as Parkinson's and Huntington's disease.[30] Resveratrol assists in creating a situation where good chemical processes flourish, while at the same time bad processes are limited. However, this only occurs to a certain extent, and the effects are not lasting. Thus, there are still a lot of unknowns in this process. In addition, though certain chemical reactions can be kept in check as a result of this positive reaction, there are often a multitude of bad things that happen on a cellular level that contribute to neurodegenerative progression. This research is another piece of the puzzle, and it will contribute to unraveling these diseases. Knowing that positive benefits have been observed in these neurodegenerative conditions with the presence of resveratrol in and of itself may provide good clues to researchers as they move forward.

As stated earlier, we know that a good diet is important for maintaining one's health, but almost as important is a well-controlled diet. Many individuals believe that if they eat their daily requirements of fruits and vegetables, this should be sufficient in providing good overall health. However, though they might meet their daily fruit and vegetable requirements, they may also indulge in high-caloric behavior, which can be detrimental to your brain. Researchers have shown that placing rats and mice on a 30 percent less caloric diet extended the lifespan of the rats and mice by 30 to 40 percent. In addition, in comparison to rats and mice who were permitted to eat at will, those on calorie restrictions demonstrated greater ability to suppress the effects of oxidative stress.[31] Caloric restriction is the only technique that has consistently been shown to slow the aging process and maintain health and vitality. A large-scale study conducted by the National Institute of Aging using primates (rhesus and squirrel monkeys) has shown a number of positive benefits. For example, separate projects showed reductions in fat mass, body weight, cholesterol, triglyceride levels, as well as arterial stiffness. This research noted that over time it is expected that these animals are less likely to experience cardiovascular disease, cancer, diabetes, and other aging pathologies.[32] However, the drawback of this research lies in the ability of individuals to reduce their caloric intake by 30 percent. To reap these benefits, individuals would need to substantially alter their eating behaviors.

Population studies have provided us with some perhaps overreaching conclusions but nevertheless are very interesting. An example of this is the comparison of societies as wholes. For instance, individuals in China and Japan on average take in 1,600 to 2,000 calories a day (a diet based on fish and rice). This is compared to the United States and Western Europe, where the average calorie intake is 2,500 to 3,000 a day. AD is also greater in the United States and Western Europe. Though this is just a casual link, it is one that continues to receive much attention.[33] It is also important to note that AD is just one of a number of neurological diseases that is reduced with reduced caloric intake.

EXERCISE

Staying physically active can maintain and enhance cognition and brain function. The following section will outline the importance of exercise and how it promotes positive brain functioning.

A fundamental question is this: is exercise an essential factor in maintaining a healthy brain as well as a healthy body? Couch potatoes, brace yourselves! Because here comes the message one more time, one we have all heard our whole lives. Yes, exercise is an essential factor in maintaining a healthy brain and body. However, this does not mean you need to train for a marathon. In fact, results from several studies suggest that even a moderate amount of activity can be beneficial to your body and your brain. The next section provides some examples of activities one should engage in and the improvements that result.

Some of the important questions asked about cognitive decline as individuals age are these: Are there things I can do to prevent this from happening to me? If it does happen to me, are there things I can and should do to slow the process? For example, if I am diagnosed with a neurodegenerative condition such as AD, is there any point to starting an exercise program? This information is much sought after because individuals and families want to know what they should do in advance of such an illness, and they also want to know what they should do in the wake of a condition becoming a reality. Let's look at some of the research.

In response to the first question, the answer is yes. There are a number of studies showing that, in fact, we all have the ability, through exercise, to reduce cognitive deficits. One such study showed significant improvements in communication skills when individuals engaged in a walking program of as little as thirty minutes a day, three times a week, for ten weeks (controlling for cardiovascular risk factors).[34] Improvements were also observed in areas such as executive functioning (planning and reasoning activities) and general cognitive functioning with a program that again required thirty minutes a day of walking or just completing modified hand or face exercises (used for individuals with limited mobility) three times a week for six weeks. Results for these programs showed significant improvements could be had compared to a control group that solely engaged in conversation activities.[35] Additional studies have shown significant general cognitive improvements when subjects engaged in activities such as bingo (daily for twenty minutes)[36] or walking and riding exercise bikes.[37] Both walking speed and distance can be associated with a reduced likelihood of experiencing AD symptoms.[38] The beneficial effects of regular physical activity as a "protective" element against the onset of dementia have been noted in fairly large research studies. In one study, 158 of 1,740 participants over the age of sixty-five developed AD. However, when adjusted for age, sex, and medical condition, individuals engaging in exercise three or more times a week were 34 percent less likely to be diagnosed with dementia.[39] Further evidence indicates that increased cerebral blood volume, which mirrors increases in cognitive performance, can be linked to increases in physical activity.[40] Once again, not only is physical activity linked to increases in behavioral measures (better test scores), but brain changes are readily visible (increased blood flow throughout the brain). Thus, even moderate rates of activity can be important for preventing cognitive decline as we age. As well, the amount of activity is shown to influence protective elements of good brain health, with subsequent benefits to overall health. Therefore, the results clearly indicate that as we age, sustained and regular exercise is an excellent way to prevent cognitive decline.

The other question put forth was whether one can disrupt the progress of cognitive decline once it has started. Again, the good news here is yes!

One of the best ways to test the effects of cognitive improvement in the face of AD has been through the use of mice models. Mice models are effective in that researchers have the ability to create animals that show consistency in AD pathology in addition to consistent ways to measure memory improvements using standardized testing environments. What the researchers found was that cognitive improvements could be seen in animals with AD pathology and that exercise was beneficial to improved thought processing even when it was started after the onset of AD.[41] The group that seemed to benefit the most, in fact, was animals that were not very active to begin with, suggesting that it is even more important for individuals with limited exposure to exercise to begin a program after a dementia diagnosis in an effort to combat the disease. Research with humans has displayed similar results. A review of numerous studies conducted between 1970 and 2003 displayed that physical training (exercise) was effective in improving not only cognitive function in individuals with dementia but also physical fitness, functional activities (e.g., preparing a meal for oneself), and behavioral measures (e.g., mood). So, to sum up, one can see that exercise has benefits at any stage of aging, including before dementia and while experiencing a dementia-related disturbance.

After reading these research results, it seems inevitable that if you want to avoid AD, you need to start being active. And quite possibly many of you have put this book down and headed out the door for a walk before getting to this section! Though I fully support the role of an active lifestyle to reduce one's susceptibility to AD, the additional benefits of reductions in stress, cardiovascular fitness, disease prevention (heart disease, stroke), increased nerve growth, weight control, sleep benefits, increased energy levels, mood improvements—the list goes on and on—deserve close attention too. However, this research needs to be tempered by the fact that engaging in a regular exercise program does not guarantee you will be spared from any major illness. Other studies fail to show that being physically active necessarily means one is less susceptible to cognitive decline.[42] But overall, there is very convincing evidence that engaging in some level of physical activity can reduce one's chances of cognitive decline. In addition to all the other benefits associated with a regular fitness program (any type of activity that challenges your current level of activity), doing nothing results in nothing being done. It is like the saying "you can't win if you don't play," except the game you are playing in this case is fairly important—your health and perhaps your life.

Now hold on before you head for the door again. Make sure your fitness level is assessed by a health-care professional, particularly before you start any regular program or you have not been active for a while. Keep in mind that consistency is very important. Set goals and a schedule that is obtainable to start off with, and then increase your goals from there if you deem it is necessary. If you require extra motivation, it is always good to get a partner, friend, neighbor, or anyone else to come with you. This can provide you with support and motivation to stay on track, especially on days when you lack that get-up-and-go. I realize the simplicity in this advice, but it really is as simple as that: increase physical activity, and you can create a number of benefits for your health. This does not mean that you need to spend a significant amount of time training; anything is better than nothing. Be aware that as you age, physical exercise is an important part of having a healthy brain. In addition, starting a regular program (whether you are fifty or ninety) can be habit forming even in your latter years, even if this has not been a focus for you to date. Remember, it is never too late to start, and you can reap the benefits within a few weeks.

EXERCISE ADVICE AND ACTIVITIES FOR BETTER HEALTH

Beginner

Endurance training (three times a week)

- 5–20 minutes of walking
- 5–15 minutes of biking (stationary is acceptable)
- 5–20 minutes of arm exercises (sitting is acceptable, standing preferred)
- 5–20 minutes of game play (e.g., lawn bowling, horseshoes, shuffleboard, bull riding [but be extra careful with this last one—maybe just watch it!])

Resistance/balance training (twice a week)

- Lift weights (use a lighter weight to begin with the first few weeks, before moving up—e.g., bicep curls, arm lifts, triceps extension)
- Leg exercises (e.g., knee flexion, hip extension, side leg raise, plantar flexion)

Stretching exercises (twice a week)

- Include your shoulders, upper arms, chest, back (lower and upper), neck, legs (back and front), thigh, hip, calf, ankle, and hamstring
- Gentle yoga

Intermediate

Endurance training (three times a week)

- 20–40 minutes of walking
- 15–35 minutes of biking (stationary is acceptable)
- 10–40 minutes of arm exercises (sitting is acceptable, standing preferred)
- 15–45 minutes of game play (e.g., tennis, golf, catch)

Resistance/balance training (three times a week)

- Lift weights (e.g., bicep curls, arm lifts, triceps extension, shoulder extension)
- Leg exercises (e.g., knee flexion, hip extension, side leg raise, plantar flexion)

Stretching exercises (twice a week)

- Include your shoulders, upper arms, chest, back (lower and upper), neck, legs (back and front), thigh, hip, calf, ankle, and hamstring
- Yoga

Sample Two-Week Programs

Table 11.1. Beginner

Week	Sunday	Monday	Tuesday	Wednesday	Thursday	Friday	Saturday
1	5-10 minute walk + stretching	Lifting weights + leg training (balance focus)	Break	5-10 minutes biking + arm exercises	Stretching or gentle yoga + weight lifting	Break	Game play
2	5-10 minute walk + stretching	Break	Weight lifting + leg training (resistance focus)	Stretching + minimum 5-10 minute walk	Break	Game play + weight lifting	Stretching or gentle yoga + leg training (balance focus)

Table 11.2.   Intermediate

Week	Sunday	Monday	Tuesday	Wednesday	Thursday	Friday	Saturday
1	20-40 minute walk + stretching or 40 minutes of yoga	Lifting weights + leg training (balance focus)	Break	15-35 minutes biking + arm exercises	Stretching + weight lifting + 25 minute walk	Break	Game play
2	5-10 minute walk + 20 minute bike and stretching	Break	Weight lifting + leg training (resistance & balance focus)	Stretching + minimum 40 minute walk + 20 arm exercises	20 minutes of biking + weight lifting	Game play or Break	Stretching + leg or 30 minutes of yoga training (balance focus)+ 30 minute walk

12

HEAD AND HEART, THE CONNECTION WE SHOULD NEVER FORGET!

After reading this chapter, you should be able to answer the following questions:

Does my chance of experiencing a dementia-related disturbance increase after having a full-blown stroke or minor stroke event?

As I age, is it normal to expect vascular issues within my brain?

Does my physical health really impact my brain health?

Is there any chance of regaining my previous level of cognitive ability after having a stroke?

If you asked experts in the field of aging what the best interventions are to stave off the effects of the aging brain, or in some cases a dementia-related illness, they would likely answer exercise, exercise, and more exercise. Exercise is the primary and by far most accessible way we can effect a change in our health. A healthy cardiovascular system is an excellent way to maintain health, not only because of the obvious benefits to our overall fitness and well-being, but also because it is an excellent way to maintain a healthy brain. In general, when we decide to go for a run, walk, or swim, we note how well we will feel afterward. And if we are consistent, our fitness level will improve and our bodies will be in better shape. However, as the last chapter clearly showed, our brain will actually benefit from these types of activities as well. In this chapter I will examine the current evidence for this heart and head connection and highlight why it is important to stay fit and active not just for our bodies but for our brains as well.

BLOOD FLOW AND THE BRAIN

When we think about cognitive impairment, we immediately wonder what is happening in the brain, and why and how impairments happen. Investigations focusing on these issues bring up all types of interesting questions. For example, is cognitive impairment a memory- or planning-based problem? If so, can we identify the specific area within the brain that is affected? Also, we might wonder how large or small of an area seems to be affected, and what regions are spared. For clinicians, it is important to examine directly what is occurring and understand where exactly something has gone wrong. These are, of course, all very logical questions to ask, and as a neuroscientist and clinical researcher I can tell you these are the focus of many studies. Possibly the bigger question to ask is, what occurred prior to something going wrong? In other words, what preexisting condition might have contributed to this current state? In recent years, there has been a greater focus on the brain's support system, including the vascular structure and why and how it may contribute to cognitive difficulties or disease. One example of how this issue has come to the forefront is through stroke research. In the case of a stroke, either the brain is deprived of proper blood flow to a certain area, or there has been a rupture resulting in bleeding in the brain. From this basic understanding, we know that disruption in blood flow creates a situation where the brain is in trouble, and in some cases it can be fatal. Therefore, we know from stroke examples that good blood flow equals a healthy brain, and problems with blood flow equal an unhealthy brain. In addition to this physiological evidence from stroke research, dementia researchers now know that vascular issues within the brain can contribute to or cause cognitive impairments.[1] In fact, over the past decade, the second most common type of dementia after Alzheimer's disease is Vascular Dementia. Recently, however, this term has evolved to encompass all related vascular and cognitive issues and is now referred to as Vascular Cognitive Impairment (VCI).[2] VCI is getting greater attention, resulting in further investigation into how this disease, and blood flow to the brain, affects cognitive ability.

VASCULAR COGNITIVE IMPAIRMENT

The clinical community appears to use the term *VCI* in favor of *vascular dementia* because it is more inclusive to various types of cognitive disruptions and impairments that occur as the result of difficulties within the vascular system. This includes attacks on the brain as a result of ministrokes (transient ischemic attacks [TIAs]),[3] full-blown strokes, or something called leukoaraiosis (white-matter hyperintensities), which is commonly defined as a vascular attack on the brain via a series of microbleeds.[4] These microbleeds are often not visible on regular CT scans and normally require a magnetic resonance imaging (MRI) evaluation to see the full extent of the damage. In fact, an MRI should be used when possible because it has better resolution on structures of the brain and can provide greater insight into the overall deficits one might be facing. Using a CT scan alone can miss areas of damage. Upon further examination, areas of concern in the brain can then be linked to cognitive deficits that have developed or may develop in the future.

I think it is important here to note that changes can occur over time and be subtle, or there might be one significant event that causes changes in an individual's cognitive performance. The problem with a subtle buildup is that cognitive change over time is not as readily recognizable to families, who often dismiss these concerns as a normal part of aging. The reason why this occurs is that family members are trying to find a way to psychologically protect themselves and their loved one from an illness that could significantly change the status quo. If there are no issues and this is normal aging, then there is no reason to be concerned and no reason to get checked out. Please keep in mind, however, that getting checked out is very important if cognition problems are impacting your daily life.

If you have a general cognitive concern and it is identified as VCI, then you have a syndrome occurring as a result of a vascular injury to the brain. As described above, this may have occurred as a result of many factors, one of which might have been a stroke, and can result in a significant change in one's cognitive ability or dementia-type impairments.[5]

VCI covers all concerns related to cognitive deficits that have developed from a vascular basis, including dementia and mild cognitive impairments that have come about as result of areas of deterioration (gaps in the brain) because of blood flow issues. When diagnosing dementia as a result of vascular concerns, there must be a deficit in performance in a minimum of two cognitive domains (such as executive/attention, memory, visuospatial ability, or language) as measured via cognitive testing. This requires prior testing, with new testing showing significant decline in at least two of the domains, and also proof that the issues are interfering with one's daily activities (imaging evidence is used when possible). Probable vascular disease is normally diagnosed when there is brain imaging evidence linked to an event (e.g., stroke) that resulted in cognitive issues, or when brain imaging shows cerebrovascular disease in an area linked to cognitive problems an individual is experiencing. This must have occurred in isolation of any history of cognitive decline.[6]

Possible vascular disease is diagnosed when one has cognitive impairment and there is evidence from brain imaging suggesting cerebrovascular disease. However, a diagnosis of possible vascular disease is used if a link between a vascular event and one's newfound cognitive impairment cannot be pinpointed; if there is not sufficient imaging evidence, despite clinical evidence, indicating a vascular issue; or if a proper cognitive assessment cannot be completed. Other issues resulting in this diagnosis are difficulty distinguishing symptoms of another neurological issue (e.g., Parkinson's or Alzheimer's disease) from those of the vascular concern, or if the individual has a history of metabolic or psychiatric disorders that have the potential to affect cognitive performance, or if cancer is involved.[7] Thus, with a diagnosis of probable or possible vascular dementia, it is important, though at times difficult, to sort out what other factors might be causing cognitive difficulties.

Vascular concerns can also mildly affect cognitive performance. Researchers have suggested a designation for such circumstances: vascular mild cognitive impairment (VaMCI). VaMCI includes amnestic (memory impairment) and nonamnestic (memory not affected) subtypes. Thus, if VaMCI includes concerns with memory, then you have the amnestic subtype; if not, then the nonamnestic subtype. However, both can include other cognitive domains or just one. Like vascular dementia, there must be evidence of a decline in cognitive ability as shown through cognitive testing. However, everyday performance of activities may or may not be affected.[8]

In the case of probable VaMCI, like vascular dementia this diagnosis will include cognitive impairment with accompanying imaging evidence of cerebrovascular disease. To receive this diagnosis, a patient will not have had a history of decline prior to some cerebrovascular event that resulted in a newfound deficit. As well, if there is clear imaging evidence in relation to a region in the brain appearing to be affected, and cognitive evidence linked to this regional deficit, you may also receive this diagnosis. Similar to vascular diagnosis, for a possible diagnosis for VaMCI, there should be no clear relationship between a cerebrovascular event and the start of a cognitive impairment, not enough or no imaging information available despite clinical symptoms suggesting VaMCI, and/or an inability to perform a proper cognitive assessment, or difficulty separating symptoms from another neurological issue. Also, if the individual has a history of metabolic or psychiatric disorders that have the potential to affect cognitive performance, then a diagnosis is difficult to make. Finally, if the individual has had or is dealing with a form of cancer, then diagnosis becomes an issue. Thus, similar to full-out vascular dementia, separating other disease states from mild vascular issues can be quite difficult and almost impossible to get a good handle on without a couple of rounds of solid neuropsychological testing and imaging evidence via an MRI.[9]

The extent of vascular involvement in the earlier stages of diseases such as Alzheimer's (or dementia) remains a key issue for researchers. Though a link between them has been known for many years, understanding how the relationship works will be of significant importance in the years to come.[10]

VCI provides researchers the ability to categorize the types of cognitive deficits being observed in the face of vascular disruptions. Individuals who have received this designation or have experienced a stroke or TIA often want to know what this means for them. They might wonder: What are the implications for my brain health as I get older? What if I have experienced a significant cerebrovascular event? What if my "brain scan" displays significant vascular issues? The following section will examine the issue related to these questions to provide a full understanding of what one could expect and what one might do in the face of these potential cognitive issues.

WHAT IS THE RISK OF DEMENTIA AFTER A CEREBROVASCULAR EVENT?

Before describing what one might typically expect in regard to vascular issues within the brain, I think it is important to review what the risk is of moving to a dementia diagnosis after experiencing a cerebrovascular event (e.g., TIA or stroke). Being diagnosed with dementia is, of course, of great concern to individuals and family members, but what, for example, is the link between stroke and dementia? In general, the risk of a dementia-related illness after having a stroke is substantially increased.[11] Of course, reports vary, but I will review some this research to provide a good understanding of what can be expected.

Researchers and clinicians who regularly deal with individuals with Alzheimer's disease examine these individuals for related vascular issues and inquire about clinical history, such as any stroke-related events. Clinicians want to understand the underlying issues and be thorough with their assessments. With imaging (e.g., MRI), they have a greater ability to locate vascular concerns such as white-matter disease and large or small silent (having occurred without the individual noticing) infarcts (strokes). Finding these issues together is becoming more and more common, and not because these events are increasing (however, there is an argument to be made that, in our growing fast food world, these issues are increasing significantly as a result of our diets), but rather the ability to detect this relationship has become much more effective in recent years.

However, getting a true understanding of the rate of this relationship is difficult in that each study carried out on this topic is quite different in how it includes individuals, the types of vascular issue (full-out stroke or TIA) being reported, or which individuals have been included for follow-up. One common theme in this research is that if one had dementia prior to a stroke, or if dementia was noted after a stroke had occurred, in both cases it resulted in an increased rate of mortality or of the individual entering a long-term care unit.[12]

Researchers have also had a great interest in understanding the timing between stroke and dementia and have examined the relative rates. Reports indicate rates of developing dementia within three months after a stroke episode ranging from 13.6 to 32 percent.[13] These percentages fluctuate depending on how the stroke episode is reported, inclusion or exclusion of certain criteria in the research (e.g., if individuals already had a cognitive impairment, there is another neurological concern, or communication was an issue for the patient, which in some studies excludes them from the research), type of stroke being examined, or other vascular factors like hypertension or arterial fibrillation (irregular heartbeat). Also, cognitive impairment as a result of a stroke can be influenced by factors such as one's level of education and age. Research has shown that younger individuals are less likely to have a significant cognitive deficit after a stroke. As well, individuals who had obtained a higher level of education were less likely to have a significant cognitive issue after a stroke, and those who are young and have higher levels of education show less long-term damage to the left side of their brain.[14] This is important because areas on the left side of the brain are primarily involved in speech and language, and damage to these areas cause significant cognitive impairment because communication is affected. As to why age and education are factors in cognitive performance, I believe this may happen for a number of reasons. As noted in a previous chapter, higher education is associated with the ability to create new pathways in the brain. These new pathways can compensate for damage within the brain and sustain neural transmission (brain messaging), meaning that your brain can still send and receive messages in spite of damage, often through the use of alternative routes. In regard to age, our brains and our bodies are designed to recover from injury regardless of any age. However, when we are younger, our brains and bodies, for numerous reasons, have the ability to heal faster. Thus, over a three-month period, we would expect younger individuals to have better scores, and they do. This does not mean that recovery to the same extent is impossible in older individuals. In fact, I believe it just takes more time, and these individuals just need to work a little harder to achieve gains and to have the same level of recovery.

Though research has focused on short periods when determining a timeline for dementia-related impairments as a result of a stroke, this research does not end at three months or six months and has followed individuals for much longer durations. A population-based study carried out over 7.3 years in the Netherlands on 6,724 individuals showed that those who experienced a stroke were twice as likely to acquire a dementia-related disease. This rate of dementia is remarkable because it occurred even when researchers removed prestroke cognitive function and decline from their analysis.[15] This means that individuals who appeared to be declining prior to having a stroke were removed from the calculation, and even when these individuals were removed the results indicated double the chance of having a dementia-related illness after a stroke event. These results are significant because they suggest that vascular issues are tied directly to one's brain health and increase the odds of being affected by a debilitating cognitive impairment. Conversely, it has also been shown that approximately 16 to 18 percent of individuals who have had a stroke already had a dementia-related illness.[16] This evidence clearly shows a relationship between vascular health and brain health at a very basic level.

TRANSIENT ISCHEMIC ATTACK AND DEMENTIA

Transient Ischemic Attack (TIA) is a difficult event to track since individuals may not always report to a health-care setting after experiencing symptoms (which are the same as in a stroke but last only a few minutes or hours). Since symptoms do not last, individuals often dismiss reporting to a hospital or their general practitioner. Thus, getting a true understanding of the long-term consequences of this type of event can be difficult to track. In addition, because a TIA is focused primarily on physical aspects, limited research has been conducted in relation to the effects TIAs have on the brain's cognitive ability, specifically as it relates to dementia. In fact, I located only one study that has tracked both acute and long-term effects related to TIA and cognitive ability over time.[17] Keep in mind that a TIA is a passing issue related to an underlying vascular problem and can result, for example, in lost or blurred vision, slurred speech, and coordination issues. These physical concerns can be quite scary, but when they resolve themselves quickly, individuals are relieved and return to normal activities. As such, people often put the incident behind them, and getting checked out may still not be a priority. In health-care settings, the focus is on the physical concerns related to this event, which are of great importance if, for example, you experience problems with your vision. However, after issues resolve, one might wonder what the lasting effects are on the brain. What can one expect concerning their cognitive ability in the days and years to come? Research on this topic has shown that individuals who experience a TIA or minor stroke show reduced cognitive ability even after physical abilities had returned, both in the short term (seven days after the event) and long term (on average, around four years later).[18] In fact, it was shown that patients with cognitive concerns seven days after a TIA or minor stroke had a five times greater chance of experiencing severe dementia than individuals who at initial assessment did not have the same level of cognitive impairment. However, at thirty days, both groups (those with and without noted cognitive issues) had similar cognitive scores, suggesting recovery to a certain extent occurred for the group that had noted cognitive deficits. Despite this recovery, as shown at the four-year follow-up, some individuals still had a significant risk of developing severe dementia. The authors of this study suggest that these results point to a subgroup of individuals who are predisposed to cognitive issues after experiencing a TIA or minor stroke, and that this group should be followed by cognitive testing to help identify ongoing concerns. Finally, this research also noted that patients presenting with initial cognitive impairments were relatively less educated and more likely to be confused during assessment.[19] These results, I believe, are quite telling, in that they directly link even minor vascular concerns with dementia. Having a five times greater risk of progressing to severe dementia in just a few years should be of significant concern to individuals who become members of this population.

In addition, researchers have also shown that the risk of dementia is increased by 33.1 percent for individuals who have a TIA within four weeks of a stroke and by 26.8 percent for individuals having a TIA more than four weeks prior to a stroke.[20] Thus, in either case, having a TIA significantly increases one's risk for developing dementia. Primary health-care institutions need to ensure that this message is being passed on to these individuals, and prevention opportunities to avoid further complications could and should be presented at that time.

HOW COMMON AND AT WHAT AGE MIGHT I HAVE A CEREBRAL INFARCTION?

First off, I will note that finding a cerebral infarct (an area of tissue loss) within in the brain of an older individual is common. Having a chronic infarct has been reported to occur in one-third to one-half of older individuals.[21] An infarct in one's brain often can be an unnoticed event. Many people have what are called silent infarcts, meaning that tissue loss has occurred in your brain but you are unaware that this has happened, simply because there were no behavioral signs to alert you. There are several physiological activities routinely carried out within the brain that we have no sense or knowledge of—for example, removing dead or dying tissue. An event such as this will go unnoticed because there are no behavioral symptoms, and thus one's performance is not affected. One of the primary questions aging individuals might have is, how common is this type of event as I age, especially if I am healthy? As I have already noted, many researchers suggest that infarcts are not all that uncommon. Healthy elderly individuals can expect to see tissue loss (lesions, infarcts) greater than the general population at a rate of 5 percent at age sixty and of 35 percent at age 90.[22] Thus, one of the mechanisms contributing to reduction in one's brain tissue is simply age.

At first glance, one might think that this is a significant concern, and that if you are in one of these age brackets you are doomed. But it is important to keep the right perspective. Though actual brain loss is certainly a great concern as one ages, the rates I have provided above are based on an average rate for a given population. They do not necessarily account for individuals who have taken great strides to protect their brain by actively engaging in weekly brain exercises (hint, hint). As has been shown, even individuals with Alzheimer's disease have the ability to alter their brain performance. It is also important to point out that the brain does not operate in isolation. If one pathway poses a problem, the brain, for example, can use twenty other pathways to transfer the same message (hence the cognitive reserve theory). The number of routes or pathways within one's brain to handle issues such as vascular disruption may depend on several factors. One factor of current interest is an individual's overall physical health. Understanding this relationship may shed some light on this connection, which I will discuss below.

Cerebral infarcts increase as one ages, but another question you might have is this: if I have one infarct, am I likely to have more? Researchers in one study tracked individuals with an average age of seventy-one (1,077 total patients, which is a good-sized sample for this type of research) over an average of 3.4 years and showed that the rate of new infarcts (silent or symptomatic) was about 14 percent, the major-ity of these (12 percent) being silent ones.[23] A factor affecting this increase was age. During the 3.4 years, individuals in the sixty to sixty-nine age group had an 8 percent infarct rate, whereas those eighty to ninety had a 22 percent rate. Women had a higher incident rate than men, but it was only slightly higher and was not significantly different. Thus, women can be assured that they did not outperform men, which in this case at least is a really good thing. Interestingly, the researchers also noted that those who had experienced a previous cerebral infarct had a 2.9 times increased chance of experiencing another. This was maintained at a rate of 2.6 when controlled for other health factors, such as hypertension, diabetes, and arterial fibrillation. This means that though one may have an additional health concern, having an initial cerebral vascular issue seems to be the best predictor that you will experience another. However, most cardiovascular risk factors for stroke in general (e.g., hypertension, smoking, diabetes) also increase the initial risk of any type of cerebral infarct.[24]

What might be important to note here is that many vascular issues that occurred in the brain in this representative population were the result of silent infarcts. This means that unless you were being tracked and given a routine MRI, you could experience many silent brain in-farcts and be totally unaware of it. This suggests the importance of engaging in good habits regardless of any physical signs you may or may not receive from your body, particularly as you age.

However, if you become aware of issues or if you have experienced an overt event like a stroke, your might wonder, can I regain my same level of cognitive ability? First and foremost, this is a difficult question to answer directly since no two strokes are alike. Two common types of stroke that affect the brain in different ways include ischemic and hemorrhagic. One of these restricts blood flow (ischemic) and the other is the result of bleeding into the brain (hemorrhagic). Both are quite harmful to your brain's health, but the extent of damage can differ quite a bit depending on the type of stroke that has occurred and where and how much of the brain has been affected. All of these factors influence recovery outcomes. With this information in mind, I can safely answer the question above as both yes and no (I understand that this is not very decisive). Because there are so many variables involved in stroke recovery, including the type, size, and area of the stroke; the individual; the time it takes to get care; and so on, one cannot possibly offer a specific answer to what will happen to one's cognitive abilities as a result of a stroke. However, what I can tell you is that after having a stroke, you can expect a cognitive impairment to persist past the episode. Some researchers suggest that this occurs at a rate of about 35 percent.[25] A number of individuals will spontaneously regain cognitive ability after their stroke episode. Again, the type of ongoing disruptions can vary, and one may have anywhere from very small to significant cognitive deficits. Though researchers suggest that there are currently no great advances in cognitive training programs for stroke victims,[26] I would suggest this will change in the years to come. I believe research is making great strides in identifying the type of tasks and programs that can be cognitively helpful for individuals in the acute poststroke stages. However, as noted above, there can be a number of lingering concerns, and individuals should be aware of these and take all measures possible to beat the odds.

HEALTHY BODY, HEALTHY BRAIN?

As I stated in the introduction to this chapter, most people understand that if we exercise and work out, we can expect overall health benefits to our body. But a benefit to our brain, specifically, is not in the forefront of many people's thoughts as they engage in such pursuits, though it should be. Evidence has shown that individuals who engage in regular physical activity can expect to see cognitive benefits. Much of the early evidence on this subject suggested that the effects were tied to an increase in one's general state of arousal.[27] This means that individuals were better at certain tasks simply because they were in a heightened state of awareness as a result of some form of physical activity. An examination of several research studies indicates that cognitive performance could be improved directly after a steady-state exercise program. However, this research also showed that cognitive performance could be negatively affected during the first twenty minutes of exercise, especially if the exercise is treadmill running versus a task such as using a stationary bike. This is understandable since brain resources would be in greater use to keep one centered on a treadmill and balanced, unlike on a stationary bike. Overall, this research, which examined fifty studies, suggested that the greatest benefit to cognitive ability could be seen twenty minutes after exercise had concluded, compared to cognitive measurements taken prior to or during an exercise program.[28] Most notably, the greatest improvement in cognitive ability after an exercise program was observed on processing speed tasks (including reaction-time procedures) and in memory procedures. It is important to keep in mind that these results fluctuate depending on the type of exercise one is performing and the type of cognitive task being administered. Not all exercise is sufficient, and not all cognitive tasks have been shown to improve performance. I have simply highlighted here the ones that have shown the greatest benefit.

Though benefits can be observed, one might wonder, what's going on in the brain? If we know that certain sustained exercise programs can positively alter our cognitive performance, the question remains: how is our brain affected in a way that improves cognitive performance? First of all, our bodies view exercise as a stressor, so our brain chemistry will alter appropriately to handle the onset of this stress. However, this stressor is not the same as others (hopefully) and exercise is seen as a welcome activity by your body, and thus the concentrations of neurotransmitters that respond to stress become altered. Particularly in exercise, neurotransmitters such as noradrenaline, dopamine, 5-hydroxytryptamine (5-HT), and cortisol change concentration levels in the brain in unique ways.[29] For instance, noradrenaline and dopamine are chemicals that improve transmission of signals within the brain, and an increase in the amount of these chemicals recruited from your peripheral systems as the result of ongoing exercise can help increase the brain's signaling and subsequently improve cognitive performance. The reason other chemicals from your peripheral system do not impact your brain as well is that the blood-brain barrier (which protects our brain from harmful toxins and an overabundance of harmful chemicals) has an affinity only to certain chemicals, and these two can cross more readily than others.[30] Thus, stimulating the body's circulatory systems is one theory for why these chemicals are present in the brain and why cognition improves. In addition, these specific neurotransmitters act on regions of the brain that are important for information processing and storage. This is just one theory for why exercise may alter cognitive performance, though. The process is very complex, with many factors involved, and I have provided only a very brief and limited explanation for how our brain chemistry can be altered. Nevertheless, I believe this explanation is one of the most viable ones in that it helps explain why duration of exercise is important to changing cognitive ability, being that it takes twenty minutes or so to have chemicals move from your peripheral areas to your brain in significant quantity and to specific areas.

Finally, I would like to examine exercise research as it relates to cognitive ability in aging individuals, being that some of the earlier information I provided in this chapter focused on individuals between the ages of eighteen and thirty. A recent review article looked at eleven separate studies examining exercise programs and the resulting cognitive outcomes in healthy individuals fifty-five and older.[31] These studies varied in type of exercise, and so the reviewers examined aerobic exercise versus other types (e.g., flexibility or balance programs and strength training programs). Overall results across all studies demonstrated that aerobic exercise versus other exercise programs had a greater ability to alter cognitive performance. Specifically, aerobic programs showed a greater change in tasks such as cognitive speed, delayed memory, and visual attention. In addition, when compared to older individuals engaging in no exercise, further gains were also seen in auditory attention and motor function procedures. Interestingly, individuals who were able to increase their cardiorespiratory fitness demonstrated at the same time improvements in cognition. On the one hand, this review suggests that there were a number of cognitive functions not affected by exercise interventions, and therefore the results should be tempered. On the other hand, it also suggested that a physically active lifestyle for aging individuals can improve fitness, which in turn could positively affect cognitive abilities.

CONCLUSION

In time, as evidence grows, it will become more apparent that cardio-vascular concerns are linked to numerous cognitive and brain health issues, including diseases. In some cases, I believe the link between cardiovascular issues and vascular brain health will be significant. In addition, important factors for general cardiovascular well-being might be the same as those that ensure good vascular brain health. Thus, it may be difficult to get a clear sense of vascular health concerns since they relate to both brain and body. But this might be a good thing since researchers, clinicians, and the public in general will develop a greater appreciation for how our vascular structure is so tightly linked to brain health and that what affects the body in general may also have a signifi-cant effect on the brain. Thus, moving forward as an aging individual, good cerebrovascular health will be essential to ensuring good brain health. There is, of course, as with all examples, exceptions to this theory, but I think in general, as more evidence is presented, a clear link will become apparent. So if you wonder what you should be doing to help your brain, might I recommend exercise, exercise, and more exercise.

Below I have provided a list of common signs and symptoms for a stroke-related event. The best advice I can give if you or someone you know is experiencing any of these symptoms is to get to a health-care center as soon as possible.

The five signs of a stroke:[32]

1. Weakness—losing strength in either the arms or legs and possible numbness in the face
2. Trouble speaking—problems understanding speech or speaking and sudden confusion
3. Vision problems—trouble seeing properly
4. Headache—severe and unusual
5. Dizziness—losing balance in conjunction with these other symp-toms

Keep in mind, as noted above, that these could be short in duration. However, it is still important to get checked out quickly—time is very important in these cases.

Remembering the FAST acronym when it comes to identifying stroke symptoms can also be very helpful.[33]

F = Face

- Uneven smile
- Facial droop/numbness
- Vision disturbance

A = Arms and Legs

- Weakness
- Numbness
- Difficulty walking

S = Speech

- Slurred
- Inappropriate words
- Mute

T = Time

- Time is critical
- Call 911

Section IV

The Futuristic Brain

13

NEUROPLASTICITY AND COGNITIVE PLASTICITY

What We Should Demand from Our Brain

After reading this chapter, you should be able to answer the following questions:

What is the difference between cognitive plasticity and neuroplasticity?

What can you expect about the size of your brain as you age?

How can one communicate and move about with just a brain signal?

How to grow a bigger brain?

What are the possibilities for an artificial brain?

BRAIN PLASTICITY

Cognitive plasticity and neuroplasticity are essential elements in ensuring brain health, growth, and performance as we age. Thus, the future of your brain is linked to your ability to increase plasticity (neuro- and cognitive), through both natural and in some cases artificial processes.

Neuroplasticity is a term generally reserved for two neural processes. One of these is neurogenesis, the brain's ability to generate new neurons. The second is called synaptogenesis, the formation of new synapses (junctions between two neurons that act as their neural messaging link), which typically happen when your brain is developing but can occur throughout your lifespan. Both of these changes are referred to as cortical reorganization; they are typically a result of brain changes occurring through stimulation and can be brought on through new experiences or novel learning.

Cognitive plasticity, on the other hand, refers to an increased dependence on brain reserves (previously successful brain processes) and how they are used in cases of adaptive changes in brain activity for successful task completion. The basic idea behind this process is that the brain tries to use what is working (neural connections and areas of the brain still processing information effectively) to get around what is not working. For example, you might think of this process as similar to driving home from work and noticing that due to road construction your normal route is blocked; there is a detour you can use, which may make your drive a little longer, but you will still get home. This is not unlike what your brain does in the face of regions or neurons that have become compromised. Instead of using the normal route, the brain becomes adaptive and will work via an alternative route or process to get you what you need.

The main distinction between these processes is that neuroplasticity refers to the ability of the brain to grow and create new neurons when needed to adapt to task demands (of course, this rate varies based on the type of brain, e.g., damaged or nondamaged), and cognitive plasticity refers to the brain's ability to use alternative routes and rely on existing brain activity and patterns to meet its needs. Both of these processes are well documented and have received a significant amount of attention, but this is usually in regard to brain development, injury, or subsequent recovery, with limited research examining these processes as they relate to normal aging and age-related diseases. However, because of the increasing longevity of the population as a whole, there is a considerable interest in understanding how the brain can adapt to age-related decline and disease states.

THE AGING BRAIN

Research tells us that, on average, starting at thirty until the age of ninety, the adult brain will lose 14 percent of its gray matter volume and experience a 26 percent loss in white matter.[1] You do not need to be a neuroscientist to know that this is not good. However, this is an average evaluation, formed by examining the brains of several individuals of varying ages, and no single study has followed one specific individual, or sets of individuals, in this age group (thirty to ninety) to understand what these changes might mean on a personal level. In some cases, certain individuals might have put in place strategies to ensure better aging, while others of a similar age have done nothing. The loss of white matter can affect one's cognitive ability. For example, demyelination (loss of the sticky stuff that coats the outside of your neurons) deep within in the brain is related to reduced memory ability in older humans.[2] In addition, studies have shown that individuals with cardiovascular disease who have experienced problems with memory and planning have a reduced amount of white matter.[3] What we know is that as we age, on average, humans experience cortical loss that can affect cognitive performance beginning primarily around the age of forty.[4] However, as I have stated, this may not be the end of the story. It has been emphasized throughout this book that putting some important strategies in place can affect the brain's aging process and keep you from losing significant cognitive ability.

COGNITIVE PLASTICITY

One of the primary ways researchers have tried to evaluate age-related decline is by linking regional cortical shrinkage to behavioral deficits. To date, this has not proved to be useful. The difficulty is that some healthy individuals with no behavioral changes can have significant cortical shrinkage in a number of areas and perform normally, and sometimes even better, on certain behavioral measures.[5] For example, a shrunken entorhinal cortex (an important memory center in the temporal lobe) does not always result in observable memory loss; this is remarkable because of the essential role this area plays in memory ability, reported many times over.[6] For aging individuals, this is actually very good to know. If you remember, earlier I stated that brain shrinkage was an inevitable factor of aging. But even in the face of cortical shrinkage, and factors such as white-matter hyperintensities (vascular damage), one's brain can adapt and compensate to operate normally and efficiently.[7] The primary question is, how do these older individuals, particularly those "under attack" from cortical shrinkage or disease, adapt to ensure successful performance? The current theory offered by many researchers involved in imaging is that these individuals enact several pathways within their brain, often called overactivation, to deal with this problem.[8] These individuals automatically (keep in mind that this is an unconscious process) call on several brain resources to ensure the job gets done and may use different strategies (a conscious process) when trying to remember something of importance, such as their first kiss. It might be that they used to remember it because of where the kiss took place, and now they remember it because of whom they kissed. The point is that they still remember the kiss, but they access the information in a different way.

Overactivation of the brain is a common process observed in studies examining successful retrieval of information by aging individuals affected by a disease state. This pattern of activation is very typical of those who have demonstrated, for the most part, consistently high cognitive ability throughout their life. These individuals presumably have a superior capability to shift resources in order to complete activities than aging individuals who have consistently had less cognitive ability. Research has shown that individuals scoring low on memory tests continue to try to activate previously successful networks, in spite of issues they may have in proper retrieval of the information. Thus, these individuals consequently are shown to be less successful in memory performance than high cognitively functioning adults, who will not only try activating previous regions but new brain regions as well. In particular, the high functioning adults activate areas on both sides of the brain (bilaterally), which is in contrast to less successful adults faced with a similar task and with the newfound burden of a disease.[9] The belief is that high cognitive functioning adults have primed their brains to work on problems through numerous paths or "networks," and thus they can adapt more readily to cognitively taxing situations. Though this may be viewed as a good strategy, it is merely a way to compensate for deficits.

Optimal performance, however, is viewed as an individual who completes tasks using the fewest cognitive resources possible while achieving a high level of performance. This is typically the type of brain activation one sees in younger individuals with no deficits.[10] Additional research has also shown that, in older adults, increased activation is observed in the brain's frontal regions when dealing with the management of numerous types of tasks, such as visual perception, as well as various types of memory tasks, including retrieval and recall. This research suggests that many individuals rely on the compensatory mechanisms (cognitive plasticity) of the frontal lobe to complete various tasks, especially in the face of advancing age. Interestingly, this change appears to occur very early in the aging process, with observable changes visible, on average, before the age of fifty.[11]

The primary message that can be taken from this cognitive plasticity is that if you work to maintain cognitive ability, and engage yourself in novel learning and challenging mental activities, the greater the chance that cognitive plasticity will work to your benefit. Any impeding disruptions in your mental ability will be put off significantly longer than individuals who have not engaged in such activities or pursuits.

NEUROPLASTICITY

From a neuroscience point of view, all humans are born prematurely. What I mean by this is that the brain still requires a significant amount of time to develop and grow. When we are born, our brain only weighs about 350 grams. Though neuronal growth is somewhat limited after this time, the main objective of the brain is to establish connections between neurons and other regions, on its way to reaching a weight of 1,400 grams, which occurs in late adolescence.[12] It is quite phenomenal that we experience almost twenty years of growth, with the frontal lobe benefiting the most in the final stages of development.[13] This may explain why so many adolescents have trouble making good decisions, being that the frontal region is significantly involved in our decision-making processes and, consequently, their brains are still maturing.

Putting the growth in size issue aside, one of the primary questions researchers have been trying to understand is this: Can aging brains grow new neurons? And if so, how effective are they at this process? The quick answer is, yes, older brains can and do experience the growth of new neurons (neurogenesis). How effective this growth is appears to depend on a number of factors, which I will discuss next.

Understanding how neurogenesis happens and the biological process that occurs as a result is very exciting. However, rather than filling up a number of pages with a substantial amount of biological detail, I will simply tell you that adult neurogenesis occurs through the production of specific cell types shown to have an affinity for a specific area of the brain in the hippocampal region. This region is involved in memory processes, and these new cells need to grow and mature to become effective in aiding neurogenesis. Until recently, in the last two decades or so, the general consensus was that we do not produce new cells as adults; instead it was thought that after growth was completed (in our twenties) all the neurons we were ever going to have were presented, and afterward we were faced with an inevitable, steady decline. However, we now know that the adult brain is capable of neurogenesis and that the growth of connection areas on and to other neurons occurs through small, branchlike structures called dendritic spines.[14] With this change in thinking, new initiatives have been undertaken to study how this growth is achieved in the face of advancing age.

Researchers suggest that these newborn cells can aid in learning and memory. As well, animal studies have shown that when mice are exposed to "enriched environments" (e.g., challenging and stimulating tasks), they demonstrate better ability in completing various tasks later in life, but in particular those related to environments they were exposed to in their early stages of neural growth.[15] This is interesting because it suggests that one can recover functions much better having been previously exposed to them during the growth stage. Providing enriched environments as one grows could be significantly important in the production of neurons in adulthood.[16] For example, many people who are exposed to a specific type of task during childhood are surprised to find they can still perform this type of task years later, even if they have not attempted it since childhood. Not only are enriched environments important as one matures, but research with mice indicates they play a role in promoting the survival of new neurons in older animals.[17] Thus, one should strive to ensure that environments are rich with activities that continually challenge and inspire the brain. As well, engaging in these behaviors in the later stages of your life will help ensure the survival of newly generated neurons and help you develop to your fullest potential.

Though preferential treatment can occur for neurons that have had an "enriched" development phase, engaging in novel tasks is also beneficial for the expression of these cells.[18] Theoretical models suggest that new neurons need time to grow and create effective connections with other neurons. The phrase "practice makes perfect" comes to mind, because, on a cellular level, this could actually be the case in the development of new neurons. Think about a person trying to make a sports team. The "new guy" is trying to fit in and find a place on the team where he works best. If there is not a good fit, the process goes on without him. However, if there is a good fit, then the team gets that much better.

It is also important to note that neurogenesis could be viewed as a process whereby these new neurons are used to compensate for neurons that are dysfunctional. Thus, a replacement process is essential for continued performance.[19] One interesting finding is that neurogenesis occurs in brain structures (e.g., the substantia nigra) noted to be affected, for example, by Parkinson's disease. Reports suggest that neurons in this area are being replaced, although this replacement is at a rate slower than the progression of the disease. The brain is working remarkably hard in attempting to defend itself and ensure successful functioning, even in the face of a neurodegenerative condition such as Parkinson's.[20]

Though research has shown that adult neurogenesis does occur, and that behavioral changes in memory and learning are possible, none of the research is entirely conclusive, and some of what is presented is based on theoretical models only. However, this simply tells us that more research needs to be conducted in order to understand how to create effective neurogenesis and fight disease in aging individuals.

BRAIN MAINTENANCE

Maintaining brain health is of the upmost importance. As noted thus far, there are several ways one can improve the chances of successful cognitive aging. Scaffolding theory has been suggested to explain how certain aging individuals are able to maintain a higher level of functioning despite changes in the brain. Scaffolding theory suggests that healthy adaptations of brain functioning occurs not just because the brain develops and creates ways to handle new challenges, but because individuals who have consistently challenged themselves throughout their lives can be very adaptive in handling changes that occur on an anatomical level at a later stage of life.[21] Individuals who continuously engage in novel activities may create a scaffold (or platform) of primed neurons, and possibly a primed neural network as well, ready to address cognitively challenging situations as they age. Secondary networks of neurons called into action with particularly challenging tasks might be used later to handle situations where the primary pathway is not functioning at an optimal level.[22] For example, neurobiological challenges (e.g., attack from diseases causing a loss of neurons) could result in limited behavioral disruption in task performance when a "scaffold" is in place; one could recruit previously established resources to ensure normal brain functioning and normal behavioral responses. It is important to note that this theory is not yet biologically established but is suggested to address why certain individuals at postmortem examination have substantial neural loss but still presented as cognitively normal to the end (a good goal for many to achieve).

As we age, there is a common tendency for the brain outside of the frontal lobe to be underactivated and the frontal area to become overactive, influencing how one adapts to cognitive challenges.[23] Interestingly, brains in younger individuals working on a complex problem resemble those of older individuals working on a simple problem.[24] Though plasticity is a possibility throughout our lives, age-related decline is a challenge and an area of concern; thus increasing our plasticity as a protective mechanism against neurological diseases could be very important for ensuring normal functioning. However, there may be a limit to the "scaffolding" system; at a certain point, compensation is not viable anymore, and this is when cognitive decline may become very apparent.[25] Many families report that their loved one seemed fine and was coping well, and then there seemed to be a sudden decline in cognitive ability, a process I postulate might be more common in individuals with a good scaffold.

COMMUNICATION AND THE BRAIN

What does the future of the brain hold for communications? Will we eventually have these wonderful superpowers, like the supreme beings we see in movies who communicate telepathically with one another? Though this seems very far-fetched, in reality communication simply requires the ability to transfer signals or information from one area to another. Thus, with the help of technology, it may be possible to transfer neural correlates of language into a system that produces an output, or response, for another individual. This means that if a person cannot speak, there could be a way to communicate through technology of some kind. Though this is not telepathy in the purest sense, it is certainly a remarkable advancement. Though you may think this is a newfound scientific achievement, people have been successfully using this type of technology for some time. Perhaps you have heard of the remarkable Professor Stephen Hawking (director of research at the Centre for Theoretical Cosmology at Cambridge). Professor Hawking uses tiny muscle movements to talk, write, and stay mobile.[26] He retains the ability to use muscle movements, which actually exceeds what many others experience, for example, muscle movements are not available in locked-in syndrome.

Locked-in syndrome, in a majority of cases, results from a brainstem stroke (vascular) and creates a situation where an individual is almost completely paralyzed. For many years, health professionals wondered if this was a vegetative state or if this individual could still comprehend what was going on around them. The question is, how can these individuals possibly communicate? One way that has been successful is through the simple efforts of blinking their eyes; and, in fact, Jean-Dominique Bauby published an entire book, *The Diving Bell and the Butterfly*, by blinking the alphabet with his left eye.[27] Discovering that these individuals are cognitively intact, and not in a vegetative state, has helped increase the research being conducted in this area. Because muscle responses cannot be used or accessed for these individuals, researchers went directly to the source: the brain. In a study at Cambridge, an individual diagnosed as being in a vegetative state (temporarily) was examined using brain imaging (fMRI), allowing the individual the opportunity to respond to questions.[28] The researchers had the individual think of two specific types of activities and equate one of them with a yes response and the other with a no. When the individual wanted to say yes, he or she would think of this identified "yes activity," and when it was "no," of the other activity. They found that the individual was able to communicate via this thought process and identify, for example, the names of his or her family members; these specific responses showed researchers that communication using just one's thoughts is possible. In a follow-up to this experiment, Dr. Owen, the lead researcher in this study, suggested that it may also be possible to use brain signals to communicate yes and no output such as seen in the scanner. However, generating a brain signal and having it identify a specific activity takes a bit of time, making a real-time conversation as it stands now difficult.[29] Despite the drawback of a lag in conversation time, it is certainly remarkable to think that we can use our brain responses as a way of communication, with no speech or muscle movement required. How this can help individuals with various diseases affecting communication will be watched closely for future developments.

BRAIN, MOVEMENT, AND BIOFEEDBACK

In the above discussion, I described how technology has evolved to address communication issues related to a breakdown in our bodies' abilities to communicate. As shown, remarkable advances have been made in this field of research. But how about our ability to move objects with our minds (telekinesis)? Could this be possible as well? This is, again, an example of extraordinary superpowers noted in popular literature and glorified in movies that could really happen in the future. Since this has not occurred yet, scientists have been developing ways that computers can interact to meet the needs of individuals who could benefit from telekinetic-like superpowers.

Current technology has shown that we have the ability to design a number of highly advanced systems that work through a process called biofeedback. Biofeedback is a process whereby an individual uses internal signals (e.g., brain or muscle activity patterns) to control external objects or improve internal functioning. The goal of biofeedback is to give the user the ability to understand, control, or modify internal responses for internal improvement or external gain. Modifying internal processes can be seen, for example, when individuals can visibly track biological processes such as their pulse or blood pressure. When given the opportunity to monitor their blood pressure or pulse, individuals demonstrate a good ability to alter and manipulate it, indicating that the brain plays a definitive role in the process.[30]

Research on this topic is exciting because it demonstrates that one can change existing internal states, but how about controlling external "things" in our world? One of the most compelling ways biofeedback has been used is to control external objects using internal thoughts or biological signals. A recent way this has been achieved is through a process called brain computer interface (BCI). BCI works by transmitting neurological signals to a computer, which then translates these signals to control some form of external device. These neurological signals can be captured via electrical brain signals or through brain blood flow; either of these types of measurements indicates activity within a certain region of the brain. Thus, in order for individuals to create an external movement, such as moving a wheelchair left or right, researchers program the computer to turn left when a particular area of the brain becomes active or turn right when a different area becomes active. Though this may sound simple, individuals trying to use this technology are required to practice activating regions for control of the device, which can be time consuming.[31] The individual thinks normally about something specific and nothing else; with this equipment, they are using their thoughts to control devices in the world around them. With these types of systems, individuals can control many items around them, such as the temperature of the room or whether the blinds are opened or closed.[32] In other examples, individuals control prosthetic devices.[33] Providing individuals that have lost an appendage with a device to allow them to grasp and move objects with a thought is of significant benefit and now possible with these recent advancements.

So how far can these types of devices go? It is difficult to say, but the future seems bright. One example comes from a company called Emotiv that has developed a system to control one's computer through thoughts. In fact, there are many demonstrations of this technology on the web, showing individuals controlling items on a computer screen. The company markets a headset device that requires no significant setup. Individuals simply place this device over their head, connect sensors on certain parts of the head (over specific regions of the brain), and then begin to calibrate the system. As the company demonstrates, individuals need to think, for example, of moving an object during the calibration phase, which allows the computer to measure signal strength and activation. The individual can then try this task with a virtual object on a screen to see if movement can be achieved. The company currently provides a number of games individuals can play through this type of thought-controlled device.[34] This is certainly a remarkable advancement that could fit nicely with a smart home system. Individuals with significant restrictions could, through a system like this one, control many of the devices in their home with just a thought. Or, as mentioned above, a person who has lost control of a limb could experience movement once again. These systems will work well if your brain is working well, but what about the brain itself? Is there a way to effect positive change or to artificially protect our brains as we age? The following section will examine some ways we might cheat the process of an aging brain.

CAN OUR BRAIN LIVE AT ITS PEAK PERFORMANCE FOR THE DURATION OF OUR LIFE?

The majority of this book has been spent explaining ways to protect your brain because, as noted, it is susceptible to so many things. Therefore, I thought it only fair to examine some ways we might cheat some of the processes affecting the aging brain. We know that as we age our brain shrinks as a result of dying tissue and neuronal loss. This is a significant concern even for healthy individuals. But is there a way to alter this process? I will review this "brain shrinkage" problem and provide some plausible suggestions.

THE SHRINKING BRAIN

Is it possible to artificially stop our brains from shrinking? One of the key components involved in the shrinkage of our brain is the reduction of the ability to produce new neurons (neurogenesis).[35] This results in ongoing loss of the formation of new brain connections and maintenance of current brain structures (e.g., in the hippocampus), causing actual physical shrinkage in your cortical brain matter. New neurons are formed with the assistance of neural stem cells. Currently, animal research has shown that we can produce neural stem cells that can flourish and grow when implanted into the brain, and this can occur even in areas with significant damage. These cells have the ability to stimulate growth in tissue that has died or experienced trauma.[36] This is very exciting news, and one might hope that issues related to disease or damage can be solved as a result of this scientific advancement. However, there is an important issue with these new cells. Because they are entering the brain without experience, they are able to create new growth and connections among each other, but they have difficulty generating connections with the existing brain structure, and thus in many cases they do not become useful. In addition, in the case of neurodegenerative diseases (e.g., Alzheimer's and Parkinson's diseases), these new neurons are still susceptible to the same disease process that has been occurring in the individual's brain for a number of years. Thus, replacing dead and dying neurons could be a never-ending process. But what if this could be changed? What if neural stem cells could undergo a maturation process before being implanted into one's brain?

The above ideas are certainly plausible; finding a way to make them work is the next step. Before understanding how to engineer new cells, it must first be determined if increased neuron density can be achieved at all, assuming that greater neuron density will ensure maintenance of brain size.

INCREASING OUR BRAINS

Researchers have indeed shown in animal models that it is possible to significantly increase neuron density, and they have successfully done so in the brains of animals that have experienced damage. It has also been shown that these new neurons could survive and mature, replicating the performance of the pervious neurons in this area, including behavioral performance on motor tasks.[37] This current research is remarkable; if it can be extended to human brain conditions, there could be a whole new approach to recovery. However, stem cells involved in this process develop into neurons that also age. Thus, if we are going to cheat the aging brain process, we need to find a way to keep these neurons young.

As we age, our stem cells mature and develop into a "required cell." These cells are provided at specific times and places. This process occurs from birth, and each successive new generation of cells, especially in the early stages, alters and changes to meet the needs of our environment and ensure growth. The goal, of course, is continued renewal of these cells, to ensure stability in health and in the genome (genetics).[38] However, the majority of the human brain does not produce or renew cells. Even though you might modify stem cells to interact with tissues to create a more youthful cell, it might not be helpful to our aging brains. Studies do, however, suggest that, on a basic level, cells from the skin, muscle, and bone marrow of a young animal can be introduced into an aging animal's genetic makeup, creating a hybrid of both, suggesting improvement for the aging animal on a cellular level.[39] If this process could be modified to meet the needs of the brain, we might reduce the number of aging brain cells and stave off cell death.

Another suggestion to fight loss of neuron density and create, in a sense, a neuroprotective effect has been examined in cases of brain trauma and stroke. Researchers have shown that, after damaging the parietal lobe of a mouse's brain, they can successfully increase neurogenic growth during recovery, as well as protect other areas of the brain around the damage site using erythropoietin (EPO). These animals were shown to regain cognitive abilities that had been impaired by brain damage. Researchers also made a very interesting observation; they suggested that discrete damage to only the parietal lobe in animals during the development stage is linked to global neurodegeneration, and can be linked to premature aging and genetic events such as Alzheimer's disease and schizophrenia. They suggest that with the treatment of EPO, these events could be avoided.[40] EPO is helpful because it protects tissue, particularly in low oxygen states. It is primarily described as a hormone for the production of red blood cells. Thus, EPO could be helpful in maintaining and regaining structural brain stability. To my knowledge, there have been no experiments examining this potential in human patients, but it may prove useful in the years to come.

An additional observation made by these same researchers was that the parietal lobe appears to be relatively important in achieving an overall healthy brain state. Thus, increasing neuron density in the parietal lobe might be very useful. Targeting specific brain regions might be achieved through substances like epidermal growth factor (EGF). To a certain extent, this process has been successful in increasing the number of new cells. Maintaining this growth and ensuring its success will be the obstacle to overcome.

Targeting the parietal lobe for growth could be important because, as already noted, it is responsible for combining information and transmitting messages to several other brain regions. It also maintains significant connections to all other brain regions via a set of fiber tracts. An interesting anecdote about the parietal lobe is that on postmortem examination, Albert Einstein was reported to have had an enlarged parietal lobe. Whether this was the mechanism responsible for his great mind no one can say for certain, but greater density certainly wasn't a drawback in his case, and might indicate better brain health, especially as we age.

ELECTRICAL CELLS

Thus far in this chapter, a number of theories have been proposed suggesting that there is a possibility for humans to ensure better brain health, and health in general, as we age. Many of the processes described here are on the cusp of great breakthroughs. Ensuring longevity requires work on a cellular level, but if a key to cell renewal cannot be provided at this point in time, then perhaps the key is in ensuring proper maintenance or, more appropriately, enhancement of cells. One of the major desires expressed by aging individuals is to have the same cognitive capacity they once did, and even perhaps the same memory ability. Could there be a way to artificially enhance neurons, and subsequently the brain structures, to get them to respond as they once did or perform even better? Recent research suggests that this is certainly a possibility and proposes a "neural prosthesis." For example, researchers conducted a study where they recorded the electrical signals within the hippocampal region of rats performing a task that required them to press the correct level to get water. Researchers successfully recorded the pattern of electrical signals that were active in forming the memory of the correct level at both the input stage (recognizing the task) and the output stage (performing correct motor movement and choice). A drug was then administered to erase the rats' memory of this activity, and researchers applied the same pattern of electrical signals to the same brain structures observed in the recording stage. They were successful in having a rat who did not remember this training act as a trained rat.[41] Thus, they showed that we have the ability to record input patterns within a brain, predict what the output pattern should be, and do this successfully to generate an appropriate behavioral response.

This research is remarkable and could be invaluable for humans. Areas affected by disease or trauma might benefit greatly from this form of artificial stimulation, providing one with the ability to complete a desired behavioral response with the use of an artificially implanted electric signaling device. As well, a reduction in cognitive performance as we age might not need to take place, and where identified structural reductions occur, electrical stimulation could fill this void.

ENHANCING OUR BRAINS

Neural implants are a current reality, and, as was highlighted earlier, brain computer interfaces demonstrate that biology and computers can already interact at a high level. This leads to the question, could more be achieved?

One of the plausible ways to enhance our brain capacity is through the development of an artificial brain. As recently as 2000, this was an arguable concept; researchers wondered whether a supercomputer could even meet the capacity (e.g., speed) of the human brain. At that time, computers were operating at rate of one hundred trillion (10^{14}) calculations per second (CPS); the goal for scientists in 2000 was to reach a rate of 10^{16} CPS by 2020, which was thought to be similar to the ability of the human brain.[42] However, this ability has progressed far beyond this initial projection, and supercomputers are measured to operate in quadrillions of CPS, with the newest models able to conduct ten quadrillion CPS (10^{16}). Furthermore, speeds are currently projected to be in the quintillion range by 2019.[43]

Since the required computing needs have been achieved, one could argue that the hardware issue is solved; what remains unsolved, however, is how to program human intelligence. As Kurzweil states, we need to "reverse-engineer the human brain."[44] This will require intimate detail of all the human brain structures and their connections. Fortunately, we have also significantly increased our ability to image the human brain, with greater spatial and temporal resolution available each passing year. In fact, research can actually image the firing of individual neurons and track interneuron connections related to specific tasks.[45] We know so much more about brain structures, and the various connections within the brain, than we did just a few years ago. In addition to this, computational models of several brain regions have been developed, including an understanding of abundant secondary neural connections. These models can simulate both electrical and chemical processes, similar to how neurons fire and how the brain operates.[46] With all this information, now is the time to try building biologically accurate artificial brain models, which would undoubtedly be useful in examining many conditions related to brain function and dysfunction.[47]

One of the great advances in building a replica of the human brain has come from a program called the blue brain project in the United Kingdom. This project has strived to build anatomically correct brain models down to the neuron level. The researchers have reported the ability to stimulate ten thousand neurons and ten million synapses using a supercomputer. The key, they believe, is in understanding the biological rules of the brain and using this as a model to develop neurons and neural connections that will respond in "natural" ways. If this brain is constructed correctly, the researchers believe then that some "brain" process will eventually happen without programming requirements. This is very exciting and will have a significant impact on our ability to reduce the two trillion dollars' worth (in Western countries alone) of health-care problems associated with brain functioning. However, despite these current advances, these researchers believe they are still ten years away from developing a whole model of the human brain, and that these years will only begin when the proper level of funding for the project is reached. The current goal is to have a workable human brain model by 2023 or 2024.[48]

If you can imagine for a moment that these needs are met (and many more not described in creating a true model), and a "human artificial brain" is developed, what might the possibilities be? Some individuals already have computer chips directly implanted into their brains; these chips interact on a neuronal level. These individuals also have the ability to download upgrades right into these chips, and thus right into their brain. These interactions occur in a computer-to-biology-based system in which the brain, a biological organism, is able to communicate with the computer, a nonbiological system. With this information, if we accept that we can develop an implicit understanding of all human brain structures, we should then be able to interact with each brain structure individually. For example, if our hippocampus (the memory center of the brain) becomes faulty, perhaps we could hook up an external hippocampus. This system could be highly interactive, and if there was a breakdown in the biological hippocampus, we would be able to back it up with an artificial one. We could also add information directly into this external memory for use in our biological brain, or download a set of encyclopedias directly into your brain. These are just some examples of the possibilities, and wrapping your mind around this concept is almost too much to comprehend, but imagining is often the first step.

What if we also had the ability to "download" our own information and experiences into a computerized system? This could essentially provide people with the ability to transmit the essence of who we are into a set of files. This computerized system could hold all our experiences and innermost thoughts, which would provide it with a framework to continuously respond to new situations based on our past performance. Therefore, this system would become an extension of "us" and, by default, a backup version of "you." To take this even one step further, if you could transmit this knowledge and experience into a cyber organism, then theoretically you could generate a computerized copy of yourself, which you might call your "cyber buddy." This cyber buddy would have the ability to respond to requests or questions in a manner similar to you because it would contain your thoughts and your experiences. This concept is certainly "out there," but the technology exists, as well as the possibility to put all of these elements together.

However, if there is no interest in living on as a "cyber buddy," and there is a desire to be "you" as long as you can be, remember to find the path that works best for you. Develop a plan, seek out the right information, and have a goal to ensure great performance and good ability as you age. Finally, remember that it took time to be who you are now, so enjoy it!

APPENDIX

TANGRAM SHAPES

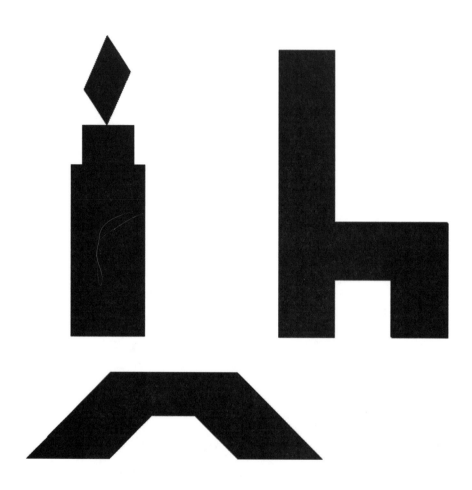

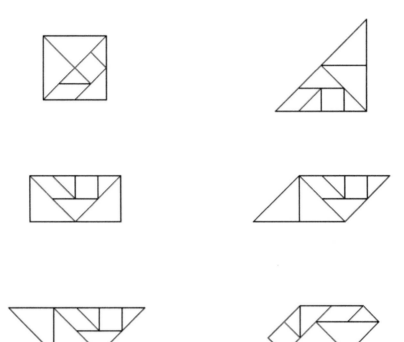

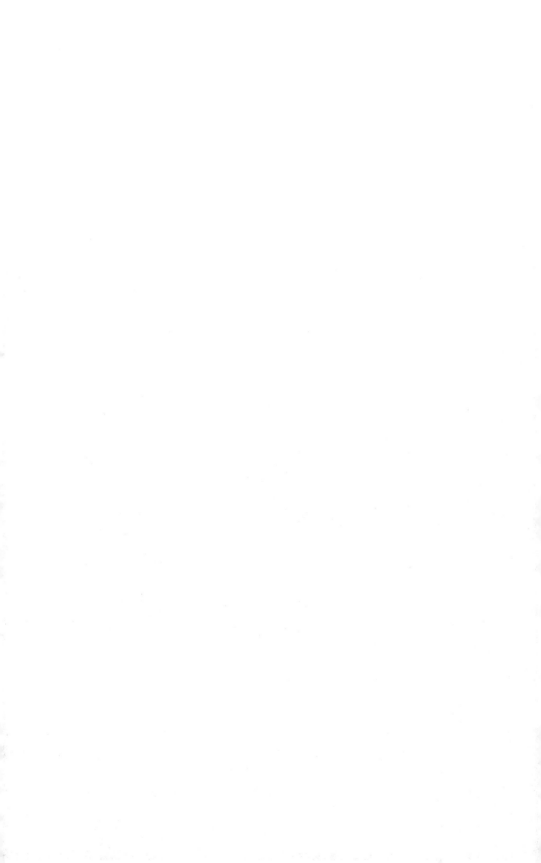

NOTES

1. THE BRAIN AGE

1. Herculano-Houzel S. The human brain in numbers: a linearly scaled-up primate brain. *Front Hum Neurosci.* 2009;3:31.

2. Harrison TM, Weintraub S, Mesulam MM, Rogalski E. Superior memory and higher cortical volumes in unusually successful cognitive aging. *Journal of the International Neuropsychological Society.* 2012;18:1–5.

3. Ibid.

4. Ibid.

5. Czaja S, Lee C. The impact of aging on access to technology. *Universal Access in the Information Society.* April 1, 2007;5(4):341–49.

6. Cheek P, Nikpour L, Nowlin HD. Aging well with smart technology. *Nurs Adm Q.* October 2005;29(4):329–38.

7. Ibid.

8. Ibid. See also Mahoney DM, Mutschler PH, Tarlow B, Liss E. Real world implementation lessons and outcomes from the Worker Interactive Networking (WIN) project: workplace-based online caregiver support and remote monitoring of elders at home. *Telemed J E Health.* April 2008;14(3):224–34; Williams K, Arthur A, Niedens M, Moushey L, Hutfles L. In-home monitoring support for dementia caregivers: a feasibility study. *Clin Nurs Res.* September 20, 2012.

9. See Bowles KH, Baugh AC. Applying research evidence to optimize telehomecare. *J Cardiovasc Nurs.* January 2007;22(1):5–15; Sirintrapun SJ, Cimic A. Dynamic nonrobotic telemicroscopy via Skype: a cost effective solution to teleconsultation. *J Pathol Inform.* 2012;3:28.

10. Svoboda E. *Smart Aging.* Toronto: Baycrest Innovation & Research; 2011.

11. Svoboda E, Richards B, Leach L, Mertens V. PDA and smartphone use by individuals with moderate-to-severe memory impairment: application of a theory-driven training programme. *Neuropsychol Rehabil.* 2012;22(3):408–27.

2. WHAT DOES THE FRONT OF MY BRAIN DO AND WHY IS IT IMPORTANT AS I AGE?

1. Carter CS, van Veen V. Anterior cingulate cortex and conflict detection: an update of theory and data. *Cogn Affect Behav Neurosci.* December 2007;7(4):367–79.

2. Dale AM, Liu AK, Fischl BR, Buckner RL, Belliveau JW, Lewine JD, Halgren E. Dynamic statistical parametric mapping: combining fMRI and MEG for high-resolution imaging of cortical activity. *Neuron.* April 2000;26(1):55–67.

3. Stuss DT, Alexander MP. Executive functions and the frontal lobes: a conceptual view. *Psychol Res.* 2000;63(3–4):289–98.

4. Jenkins LJ, Ranganath C. Prefrontal and medial temporal lobe activity at encoding predicts temporal context memory. *J Neurosci.* November 17, 2010;30(46):15558–65.

5. Hamilton AC, Martin RC, Burton PC. Converging functional magnetic resonance imaging evidence for a role of the left inferior frontal lobe in semantic retention during language comprehension. *Cogn Neuropsychol.* April 16, 2010;1–20.

6. Grindrod CM, Bilenko NY, Myers EB, Blumstein SE. The role of the left inferior frontal gyrus in implicit semantic competition and selection: an event-related fMRI study. *Brain Res.* September 10, 2008;1229:167–78.

7. Krawczyk DC, Michelle MM, Donovan CM. A hierarchy for relational reasoning in the prefrontal cortex. *Cortex.* May 2011;47(5):588–97.

8. Williamson C, Alcantar O, Rothlind J, Cahn-Weiner D, Miller BL, Rosen HJ. Standardised measurement of self-awareness deficits in FTD and AD. *J Neurol Neurosurg Psychiatry.* February 2010;81(2):140–45.

9. Carlson NR. *Physiology of Behavior.* 11th ed. Amherst: Pearson; 2013.

10. Giovagnoli AR, Erbetta A, Reati F, Bugiani O. Differential neuropsychological patterns of frontal variant frontotemporal dementia and Alzheimer's disease in a study of diagnostic concordance. *Neuropsychologia.* April 2008;46(5):1495–1504.

11. Bozeat S, Gregory CA, Ralph MA, Hodges JR. Which neuropsychiatric and behavioural features distinguish frontal and temporal variants of fronto-

temporal dementia from Alzheimer's disease? *J Neurol Neurosurg Psychiatry.* August 2000;69(2):178–86.

12. Gregory C, Lough S, Stone V, Erzinclioglu S, Martin L, Baron-Cohen S, Hodges JR. Theory of mind in patients with frontal variant frontotemporal dementia and Alzheimer's disease: theoretical and practical implications. *Brain.* April 2002;125(4):752–64.

13. Bozeat et al. Which neuropsychiatric and behavioural features? *J Neurol Neurosurg Psychiatry.*

14. Giovagnoli et al. Differential neuropsychological patterns. *Neuropsychologia.*

15. Cabeza R. Hemispheric asymmetry reduction in older adults: the HAROLD model. *Psychol Aging.* March 2002;17(1):85–100; Park DC, Reuter-Lorenz P. The adaptive brain: aging and neurocognitive scaffolding. *Annu Rev Psychol.* 2009;60:173–96.

16. Eyler LT, Sherzai A, Kaup AR, Jeste DV. A review of functional brain imaging correlates of successful cognitive aging. *Biol Psychiatry.* February 10, 2011.

17. Wolpaw JR. Brain-computer interfaces as new brain output pathways. *J Physiol.* March 15, 2007;579(3):613–19.

3. WHERE IT ALL COMES TOGETHER

1. Duhamel JR, Colby CL, Goldberg ME. The updating of the representation of visual space in parietal cortex by intended eye movements. *Science.* January 3, 1992;255(5040):90–92; Grea H, Pisella L, Rossetti Y, Desmurget M, Tilikete C, Grafton S, Prablanc C, Vighetto A. A lesion of the posterior parietal cortex disrupts on-line adjustments during aiming movements. *Neuropsychologia.* 2002;40(13):2471–80.

2. Lezak MD. *Neuropsychological Assessment.* 3rd ed. New York: Oxford University Press; 1995.

3. Benton AL. Neuropsychological assessment. *Annu Rev Psychol.* 1994;45:1–23.

4. Revill KP, Karnath HO, Rorden C. Distinct anatomy for visual search and bisection: a neuroimaging study. *Neuroimage.* May 7, 2011; Ohlendorf S, Sprenger A, Speck O, Glauche V, Haller S, Kimmig H. Visual motion, eye motion, and relative motion: a parametric fMRI study of functional specializations of smooth pursuit eye movement network areas. *J Vis.* 2010;10(14):21; Chapman HL, Eramudugolla R, Gavrilescu M, Strudwick MW, Loftus A, Cunnington R, Mattingley JB. Neural mechanisms underlying spatial realignment during adaptation to optical wedge prisms. *Neuropsychologia.* July

2010;48(9):2595–2601; Usui N, Haji T, Maruyama M, Katsuyama N, Uchida S, Hozawa A, Omori K, Tsuji I, Kawashima R, Taira M. Cortical areas related to performance of WAIS Digit Symbol Test: a functional imaging study. *Neurosci Lett.* September 29, 2009;463(1):1–5; de Vries PM, de Jong BM, Bohning DE, Walker JA, George MS, Leenders KL. Changes in cerebral activations during movement execution and imagery after parietal cortex TMS interleaved with 3T MRI. *Brain Res.* August 18, 2009;1285:58–68.

5. Cabeza R. Cognitive neuroscience of aging: contributions of functional neuroimaging. *Scand J Psychol.* July 2001;42(3):277–86; Ward NS, Frackowiak RS. Age-related changes in the neural correlates of motor performance. *Brain.* April 2003;126(4):873–88.

6. Jenkin M, Harris L. *Cortical Mechanisms of Vision.* Cambridge: Cambridge University Press; 2009.

7. Voelcker-Rehage C. Motor-skill learning in older adults: a review of studies on age-related differences. *European Review of Aging and Physical Activity.* April 2008;5(1):5–16.

8. Piefke M, Onur OA, Fink GR. Aging-related changes of neural mechanisms underlying visual-spatial working memory. *Neurobiol Aging.* December 2, 2010.

9. Gunther ML, Jackson JC, Ely EW. Loss of IQ in the ICU brain injury without the insult. *Med Hypotheses.* 2007;69(6):1179–82.

10. Nadolne MJ, Stringer AY. Ecologic validity in neuropsychological assessment: prediction of wayfinding. *J Int Neuropsychol Soc.* September 2001;7(6):675–82.

11. McCarthy RA, Evans JJ, Hodges JR. Topographic amnesia: spatial memory disorder, perceptual dysfunction, or category specific semantic memory impairment? *J Neurol Neurosurg Psychiatry.* March 1996;60(3):318–25.

4. REASONS NOT TO FORGET THE TEMPORAL LOBE AND HOW WE SEE THE OCCIPITAL LOBE

1. Carlson NR. *Physiology of Behavior.* 11th ed. Amherst: Pearson; 2013.

2. Pedersen PM, Jorgensen HS, Nakayama H, Raaschou HO, Olsen TS. Aphasia in acute stroke: incidence, determinants, and recovery. *Ann Neurol.* October 1995;38(4):659–66; Wade DT, Hewer RL, David RM, Enderby PM. Aphasia after stroke: natural history and associated deficits. *J Neurol Neurosurg Psychiatry.* January 1986;49(1):11–16.

3. McKhann G, Drachman D, Folstein M, Katzman R, Price D, Stadlan EM. Clinical diagnosis of Alzheimer's disease: report of the NINCDS-ADRDA Work Group under the auspices of Department of Health and Human

Services Task Force on Alzheimer's Disease. *Neurology.* July 1984;34(7):939–44.

4. Faber-Langendoen K, Morris JC, Knesevich JW, LaBarge E, Miller JP, Berg L. Aphasia in senile dementia of the Alzheimer type. *Ann Neurol.* April 1988;23(4):365–70.

5. Bayles KA, Tomoeda CK. Caregiver report of prevalence and appearance order of linguistic symptoms in Alzheimer's patients. *Gerontologist.* April 1991;31(2):210–16.

6. Carlson. *Physiology of Behavior*; Gazzaniga MS. *Psychological Science.* 3rd ed. New York: W. W. Norton; 2012.

7. Garrett B. *Brain & Behavior.* 3rd ed. Thousand Oaks, CA: Sage; 2011.

8. Ibid.

9. Hassabis D, Chu C, Rees G, Weiskopf N, Molyneux PD, Maguire EA. Decoding neuronal ensembles in the human hippocampus. *Curr Biol.* April 14, 2009;19(7):546–54.

10. Carlson. *Physiology of Behavior.*

11. Holroyd S, Shepherd ML, Downs JH. Occipital atrophy is associated with visual hallucinations in Alzheimer's disease. *J Neuropsychiatry Clin Neurosci.* 2000;12(1):25–28.

12. Lin SH, Yu CY, Pai MC. The occipital white matter lesions in Alzheimer's disease patients with visual hallucinations. *Clin Imaging.* November 2006;30(6):388–93.

13. Garrett B. *Brain & Behavior*; Alkire MT, Haier RJ, Fallon JH, Cahill L. Hippocampal, but not amygdala, activity at encoding correlates with long-term, free recall of nonemotional information. *Proc Natl Acad Sci USA.* November 24, 1998;95(24):14506–10.

14. Zierhut K, Bogerts B, Schott B, Fenker D, Walter M, Albrecht D, Steiner J, Schutze H, Northoff G, Duzel E, Schiltz K. The role of hippocampus dysfunction in deficient memory encoding and positive symptoms in schizophrenia. *Psychiatry Res.* September 30, 2010;183(3):187–94.

15. Parent MB, Krebs-Kraft DL, Ryan JP, Wilson JS, Harenski C, Hamann S. Glucose administration enhances fMRI brain activation and connectivity related to episodic memory encoding for neutral and emotional stimuli. *Neuropsychologia.* April 2011;49(5):1052–66.

16. Danker JF, Anderson JR. The ghosts of brain states past: remembering reactivates the brain regions engaged during encoding. *Psychol Bull.* January 2010;136(1):87–102.

17. Binder JR, Gross WL, Allendorfer JB, Bonilha L, Chapin J, Edwards JC, Grabowski TJ, Langfitt JT, Loring DW, Lowe MJ, Koenig K, Morgan PS, Ojemann JG, Rorden C, Szaflarski JP, Tivarus ME, Weaver KE. Mapping

anterior temporal lobe language areas with fMRI: a multicenter normative study. *Neuroimage.* January 15, 2011;54(2):1465–75.

18. Visser M, Lambon Ralph MA. Differential contributions of bilateral ventral anterior temporal lobe and left anterior superior temporal gyrus to semantic processes. *J Cogn Neurosci.* October 2011;23(10):3121–31.

19. Kolb B, Whishaw IQ. *Fundamentals of Human Neuropsychology.* 6th ed. New York: Worth; 2009.

20. Ibid.

21. Xu J, Kobayashi S, Yamaguchi S, Iijima K, Okada K, Yamashita K. Gender effects on age-related changes in brain structure. *AJNR Am J Neuroradiol.* January 2000;21(1):112–18.

22. Ibid.

23. Curiati PK, Tamashiro JH, Squarzoni P, Duran FL, Santos LC, Wajngarten M, Leite CC, Vallada H, Menezes PR, Scazufca M, Busatto GF, Alves TC. Brain structural variability due to aging and gender in cognitively healthy elders: results from the Sao Paulo Ageing and Health study. *Am J Neuroradiol.* November 2009;30(10):1850–56.

24. Resnick SM, Goldszal AF, Davatzikos C, Golski S, Kraut MA, Metter EJ, Bryan RN, Zonderman AB. One-year age changes in MRI brain volumes in older adults. *Cereb Cortex.* May 2000;10(5):464–72.

25. Ibid.

26. Bartzokis G, Beckson M, Lu PH, Nuechterlein KH, Edwards N, Mintz J. Age-related changes in frontal and temporal lobe volumes in men: a magnetic resonance imaging study. *Arch Gen Psychiatry.* May 2001;58(5):461–65; Bartzokis G, Cummings JL, Sultzer D, Henderson VW, Nuechterlein KH, Mintz J. White matter structural integrity in healthy aging adults and patients with Alzheimer disease: a magnetic resonance imaging study. *Arch Neurol.* March 2003;60(3):393–98; Raz N, Lindenberger U, Rodrigue KM, Kennedy KM, Head D, Williamson A, Dahle C, Gerstorf D, Acker JD. Regional brain changes in aging healthy adults: general trends, individual differences and modifiers. *Cereb Cortex.* November 2005;15(11):1676–89.

27. Bookheimer SY, Zeffiro IA, Blaxton T, Gaillard W, Theodore W. Regional cerebral blood flow during object naming and word reading. *Human Brain Mapping.* 1995;3(2):93–106.

28. Schacter DL, Curran T, Reiman EM, Chen K, Bandy DJ, Frost JT. Medial temporal lobe activation during episodic encoding and retrieval: a PET study. *Hippocampus.* 1999;9(5):575–81.

29. Dehaene-Lambertz G, Dehaene S, Hertz-Pannier L. Functional neuroimaging of speech perception in infants. *Science.* December 6, 2002;298(5600):2013–15; Pallier C, Dehaene S, Poline JB, LeBihan D, Argenti AM, Dupoux E, Mehler J. Brain imaging of language plasticity in adopted

adults: can a second language replace the first? *Cereb Cortex.* February 2003;13(2):155–61.

5. WHAT IS COGNITIVE RESERVE AND HOW IMPORTANT IS IT IN MAINTAINING A HEALTHY BRAIN?

1. Reuter-Lorenz PA, Lustig C. Brain aging: reorganizing discoveries about the aging mind. *Curr Opin Neurobiol.* April, 2005;15(2):245–51.

2. Marioni RE, van den Hout A, Valenzuela MJ, Brayne C, Matthews FE. Active cognitive lifestyle associates with cognitive recovery and a reduced risk of cognitive decline. *J Alzheimers Dis.* October 4, 2011.

3. Reuter-Lorenz, Lustig. Brain aging. *Curr Opin Neurobiol*

4. Murray AD, Staff RT, McNeil CJ, Salarirad S, Ahearn TS, Mustafa N, Whalley LJ. The balance between cognitive reserve and brain imaging biomarkers of cerebrovascular and Alzheimer's diseases. *Brain.* November 18, 2011.

5. Sole-Padulles C, Bartres-Faz D, Junque C, Vendrell P, Rami L, Clemente IC, Bosch B, Villar A, Bargallo N, Jurado MA, Barrios M, Molinuevo JL. Brain structure and function related to cognitive reserve variables in normal aging, mild cognitive impairment and Alzheimer's disease. *Neurobiol Aging.* July 2009;30(7):1114–24.

6. Schweizer TA, Ware J, Fischer CE, Craik FI, Bialystok E. Bilingualism as a contributor to cognitive reserve: evidence from brain atrophy in Alzheimer's disease. *Cortex.* April 27, 2011.

7. Bialystok E, Craik FI. Bilingualism and naming: implications for cognitive assessment. *J Int Neuropsychol Soc.* March 2007;13(2):209–11; Craik FI, Bialystok E, Freedman M. Delaying the onset of Alzheimer disease: bilingualism as a form of cognitive reserve. *Neurology.* November 9, 2010;75(19):1726–29.

8. Fritsch T, Smyth KA, McClendon MJ, Ogrocki PK, Santillan C, Larsen JD, Strauss ME. Associations between dementia/mild cognitive impairment and cognitive performance and activity levels in youth. *J Am Geriatr Soc.* July 2005;53(7):1191–96.

9. Maguire EA, Gadian DG, Johnsrude IS, Good CD, Ashburner J, Frackowiak RS, Frith CD. Navigation-related structural change in the hippocampi of taxi drivers. *Proc Natl Acad Sci USA.* April 11, 2000;97(8):4398–4403.

10. Smyth KA, Fritsch T, Cook TB, McClendon MJ, Santillan CE, Friedland RP. Worker functions and traits associated with occupations and the development of AD. *Neurology.* August 10, 2004;63(3):498–503.

11. Ibid.; Evans DA, Hebert LE, Beckett LA, Scherr PA, Albert MS, Chown MJ, Pilgrim DM, Taylor JO. Education and other measures of socioeconomic status and risk of incident Alzheimer disease in a defined population of older persons. *Arch Neurol.* November 1997;54(11):1399–1405; Stern Y, Gurland B, Tatemichi TK, Tang MX, Wilder D, Mayeux R. Influence of education and occupation on the incidence of Alzheimer's disease. *JAMA.* April 6, 1994;271(13):1004–10.

12. Fritsch T, Smyth KA, Debanne SM, Petot GJ, Friedland RP. Participation in novelty-seeking leisure activities and Alzheimer's disease. *J Geriatr Psychiatry Neurol.* September 2005;18(3):134–41.

13. Marlatt MW, Lucassen PJ. Neurogenesis and Alzheimer's disease: biology and pathophysiology in mice and men. *Curr Alzheimer Res.* March 2010;7(2):113–25.

14. Ibid.; Laplagne DA, Esposito MS, Piatti VC, Morgenstern NA, Zhao C, van Praag H, Gage FH, Schinder AF. Functional convergence of neurons generated in the developing and adult hippocampus. *PLoS Biol.* November 2006;4(12):e409.

6. ALZHEIMER'S DISEASE

1. McKhann G, Drachman D, Folstein M, Katzman R, Price D, Stadlan EM. Clinical diagnosis of Alzheimer's disease: report of the NINCDS-ADRDA Work Group under the auspices of Department of Health and Human Services Task Force on Alzheimer's Disease. *Neurology.* July 1984;34(7):939–44.

2. McKhann GM, Knopman DS, Chertkow H, Hyman BT, Jack CR, Jr., Kawas CH, Klunk WE, Koroshetz WJ, Manly JJ, Mayeux R, Mohs RC, Morris JC, Rossor MN, Scheltens P, Carrillo MC, Thies B, Weintraub S, Phelps CH. The diagnosis of dementia due to Alzheimer's disease: recommendations from the National Institute on Aging-Alzheimer's Association workgroups on diagnostic guidelines for Alzheimer's disease. *Alzheimer's Dement.* May 2011;7(3):263–69.

3. Carlson Neil R. *Physiology of Behavior.* 11th ed. Amherst: Pearson; 2013; Guardia-Laguarta C, Pera M, Lleo A. Gamma-secretase as a therapeutic target in Alzheimer's disease. *Curr Drug Targets.* April 2010;11(4):506–17; Ritchie AE. *The a1-Antichymotrypsin-51bp Promoter Polymorphism: Functional Activity and Its Role in Alzheimer's Disease* [PhD thesis]. University of Nottingham; 2004.

4. Carlson. *Physiology of Behavior*; Iqbal K, Alonso AC, Gong CX, Khatoon S, Pei JJ, Wang JZ, Grundke-Iqbal I. Mechanisms of neurofibrillary de-

generation and the formation of neurofibrillary tangles. *J Neural Transm Suppl.* 1998;53:169–80.

5. Blennow K, de Leon MJ, Zetterberg H. Alzheimer's disease. *Lancet.* July 29, 2006;368(9533):387–403; Raber J, Huang Y, Ashford JW. ApoE genotype accounts for the vast majority of AD risk and AD pathology. *Neurobiol Aging.* May 2004;25(5):641–50.

6. Blennow, de Leon, Zetterberg. Alzheimer's disease. *Lancet*; Mayeux R, Stern Y. Epidemiology of Alzheimer disease. *Cold Spring Harb Perspect Med.* 2012;2(8); Mayeux R. Epidemiology of neurodegeneration. *Annu Rev Neurosci.* 2003;26:81–104.

7. Mayeux, Stern. Epidemiology of Alzheimer disease. *Cold Spring Harb Perspect Med.*

8. Foster HD. Why the preeminent risk factor in sporadic Alzheimer's disease cannot be genetic. *Med Hypotheses.* July 2002;59(1):57–61.

9. Fan M, Liu B, Zhou Y, Zhen X, Xu C, Jiang T. Cortical thickness is associated with different apolipoprotein E genotypes in healthy elderly adults. *Neurosci Lett.* August 2010 2;479(3):332–36.

10. Levy-Lahad E, Wijsman EM, Nemens E, Anderson L, Goddard KA, Weber JL, Bird TD, Schellenberg GD. A familial Alzheimer's disease locus on chromosome 1. *Science.* August 18, 1995;269(5226):970–73; Raux G, Guyant-Marechal L, Martin C, Bou J, Penet C, Brice A, Hannequin D, Frebourg T, Campion D. Molecular diagnosis of autosomal dominant early onset Alzheimer's disease: an update. *J Med Genet.* October 2005;42(10):793–95; Rogaev EI, Sherrington R, Rogaeva EA, Levesque G, Ikeda M, Liang Y, Chi H, Lin C, Holman K, Tsuda T. Familial Alzheimer's disease in kindreds with missense mutations in a gene on chromosome 1 related to the Alzheimer's disease type 3 gene. *Nature.* August 31, 1995;376(6543):775–78; Sherrington R, Rogaev EI, Liang Y, Rogaeva EA, Levesque G, Ikeda M, Chi H, Lin C, Li G, Holman K, Tsuda T, Mar L, Foncin JF, Bruni AC, Montesi MP, Sorbi S, Rainero I, Pinessi L, Nee L, Chumakov I, Pollen D, Brookes A, Sanseau P, Polinsky RJ, Wasco W, Da Silva HA, Haines JL, Perkicak-Vance MA, Tanzi RE, Roses AD, Fraser PE, Rommens JM, St George-Hyslop PH. Cloning of a gene bearing missense mutations in early-onset familial Alzheimer's disease. *Nature.* June 29, 1995;375(6534):754–60.

11. Goedert M, Spillantini MG. A century of Alzheimer's disease. *Science.* November 3, 2006;314(5800):777–81.

12. Raux et al. Molecular diagnosis. *J Med Genet.*

13. Cruts M, van Duijn CM, Backhovens H, Van den Broeck M, Wehnert A, Serneels S, Sherrington R, Hutton M, Hardy J, St George-Hyslop PH, Hofman A, Van BC. Estimation of the genetic contribution of presenilin-1 and

-2 mutations in a population-based study of presenile Alzheimer disease. *Hum Mol Genet.* January 1998;7(1):43–51.

14. Mayeux, Stern. Epidemiology of Alzheimer disease. *Cold Spring Harb Perspect Med.*

15. Frisoni GB, Pievani M, Testa C, Sabattoli F, Bresciani L, Bonetti M, Beltramello A, Hayashi KM, Toga AW, Thompson PM. The topography of grey matter involvement in early and late onset Alzheimer's disease. *Brain.* March 2007;130(3):720–30.

16. Ikonomovic MD, Klunk WE, Abrahamson EE, Mathis CA, Price JC, Tsopelas ND, Lopresti BJ, Ziolko S, Bi W, Paljug WR, Debnath ML, Hope CE, Isanski BA, Hamilton RL, Dekosky ST. Post-mortem correlates of in vivo PiB-PET amyloid imaging in a typical case of Alzheimer's disease. *Brain.* June 2008;131(6):1630–45.

17. Jack CR, Jr., Albert MS, Knopman DS, McKhann GM, Sperling RA, Carrillo MC, Thies B, Phelps CH. Introduction to the recommendations from the National Institute on Aging–Alzheimer's Association workgroups on diagnostic guidelines for Alzheimer's disease. *Alzheimer's Dement.* May 2011;7(3):257–62.

18. McKhann et al. The diagnosis of dementia due to Alzheimer's disease. *Alzheimer's Dement.*

19. Ibid.

20. Ibid.

21. Ibid.

22. Geldmacher DS, Whitehouse PJ. Differential diagnosis of Alzheimer's disease. *Neurology.* May 1997;48(5, suppl 6):S2–S9.

23. Den Heijer T, Geerlings MI, Hoebeek FE, Hofman A, Koudstaal PJ, Breteler MM. Use of hippocampal and amygdalar volumes on magnetic resonance imaging to predict dementia in cognitively intact elderly people. *Arch Gen Psychiatry.* January 2006;63(1):57–62; Den Heijer T, Sijens PE, Prins ND, Hofman A, Koudstaal PJ, Oudkerk M, Breteler MM. MR spectroscopy of brain white matter in the prediction of dementia. *Neurology.* February 28, 2006;66(4):540–44.

24. Silverman DH, Small GW, Chang CY, Lu CS, Kung De Aburto MA, Chen W, Czernin J, Rapoport SI, Pietrini P, Alexander GE, Schapiro MB, Jagust WJ, Hoffman JM, Welsh-Bohmer KA, Alavi A, Clark CM, Salmon E, de Leon MJ, Mielke R, Cummings JL, Kowell AP, Gambhir SS, Hoh CK, Phelps ME. Positron emission tomography in evaluation of dementia: regional brain metabolism and long-term outcome. *JAMA.* November 7, 2001;286(17):2120–27.

25. Komarova NL, Thalhauser CJ. High degree of heterogeneity in Alzheimer's disease progression patterns. *PLoS Comput Biol.* November 2011;7(11):e1002251.

26. Thalhauser CJ, Komarova NL. Alzheimer's disease: rapid and slow progression. *J R Soc Interface.* January 7, 2012;9(66):119–26.

27. Kester MI, van der Vlies AE, Blankenstein MA, Pijnenburg YA, van Elk EJ, Scheltens P, van der Flier WM. CSF biomarkers predict rate of cognitive decline in Alzheimer disease. *Neurology.* October 27, 2009;73(17):1353–58.

28. Ueki A, Shinjo H, Shimode H, Nakajima T, Morita Y. Factors associated with mortality in patients with early-onset Alzheimer's disease: a five-year longitudinal study. *Int J Geriatr Psychiatry.* August 2001;16(8):810–15.

29. Komarova, Thalhauser. High degree of heterogeneity. *PLoS Comput Biol.*

30. Simonelli C, Tripodi F, Rossi R, Fabrizi A, Lembo D, Cosmi V, Pierleoni L. The influence of caregiver burden on sexual intimacy and marital satisfaction in couples with an Alzheimer spouse. *Int J Clin Pract.* January 2008;62(1):47–52.

31. Ibid.; Davies HD, Zeiss AM, Shea EA, Tinklenberg JR. Sexuality and intimacy in Alzheimer's patients and their partners. *Sexuality and Disability.* 1998;16(3):193–203; Davies HD, Sridhar SB, Newkirk LA, Beaudreau SA, O'Hara R. Gender differences in sexual behaviors of AD patients and their relationship to spousal caregiver well-being. *Aging Ment Health.* 2012;16(1):89–101.

32. Davies et al. Gender differences in sexual behaviors. *Aging Ment Health.*

33. Davies et al. Sexuality and intimacy in Alzheimer's patients. *Sexuality and Disability.*

34. Davies et al. Gender differences in sexual behaviors. *Aging Ment Health.*

35. Simonelli et al. The influence of caregiver burden on sexual intimacy. *Int J Clin Pract.*

36. Zeiss AM, Davies HD, Wood M, Tinklenberg JR. The incidence and correlates of erectile problems in patients with Alzheimer's disease. *Arch Sex Behav.* August 1990;19(4):325–31.

37. Harris SM, Adams MS, Zubatsky M, White M. A caregiver perspective of how Alzheimer's disease and related disorders affect couple intimacy. *Aging Ment Health.* November 2011; 15(8):950–60.

38. Ibid.; Davies et al. Sexuality and intimacy in Alzheimer's patients. *Sexuality and Disability.*

39. Davies et al. Sexuality and intimacy in Alzheimer's patients. *Sexuality and Disability*; Harris et al. A caregiver perspective. *Aging Ment Health.*

40. Simonelli et al. The influence of caregiver burden on sexual intimacy. *Int J Clin Pract.*

41. Fan J, Stukas S, Wong C, Chan J, May S, DeValle N, Hirsch-Reinshagen V, Wilkinson A, Oda MN, Wellington CL. An ABCA1-independent pathway for recycling a poorly lipidated 8.1 nm apolipoprotein E particle from glia. *J Lipid Res.* September 2011;52(9):1605–16; Hirsch-Reinshagen V, Zhou S, Burgess BL, Bernier L, McIsaac SA, Chan JY, Tansley GH, Cohn JS, Hayden MR, Wellington CL. Deficiency of ABCA1 impairs apolipoprotein E metabolism in brain. *J Biol Chem.* September 24, 2004;279(39):41197–41207; Wahrle SE, Jiang H, Parsadanian M, Legleiter J, Han X, Fryer JD, Kowalewski T, Holtzman DM. ABCA1 is required for normal central nervous system ApoE levels and for lipidation of astrocyte-secreted apoE. *J Biol Chem.* September 24, 2004;279(39):40987–93; Wahrle SE, Jiang H, Parsadanian M, Kim J, Li A, Knoten A, Jain S, Hirsch-Reinshagen V, Wellington CL, Bales KR, Paul SM, Holtzman DM. Overexpression of ABCA1 reduces amyloid deposition in the PDAPP mouse model of Alzheimer disease. *J Clin Invest.* February 2008;118(2):671–82.

42. Relkin N, Bettger L, Tsakanikas D, Ravdin L. Three year follow-up on the IVIG for Alzheimer's phase II study. Paper presented at: Alzheimer's Association International Conference; Tuesday, July 17, 2012; Vancouver CA; abstract P3-381.

43. Sperling R, Donohue M, Aisen P. The A4 trial: anti-amyloid treatment of asymptomatic alzheimer's disease. Paper presented at: Alzheimer's Association International Conference; Tuesday, July 17, 2012; Vancouver CA; abstract F3-04-01.

44. Reiman E, Lopera F, Langbaum J, Fleisher A, Ayutyanont N, Quiroz Y, Jakimovich L, Langlois C, Tariot P. The alzheimer's prevention initiative. Paper presented at: Alzheimer's Association International Conference; Tuesday, July 17, 2012; Vancouver CA; abstract F3-04-03.

7. CAN COGNITIVE TRAINING AFFECT THE COURSE OF AGING AND DISEASE?

1. Kennedy AM, Boyle EM, Traynor O, Walsh T, Hill AD. Video gaming enhances psychomotor skills but not visuospatial and perceptual abilities in surgical trainees. *J Surg Educ.* September 2011;68(5):414–20.

2. Lynch J, Aughwane P, Hammond TM. Video games and surgical ability: a literature review. *J Surg Educ.* May 2010;67(3):184–89.

3. Boot WR, Kramer AF, Simons DJ, Fabiani M, Gratton G. The effects of video game playing on attention, memory, and executive control. *Acta Psychol (Amst)*. November 2008;129(3):387–98.

4. Clark JE, Lanphear AK, Riddick CC. The effects of videogame playing on the response selection processing of elderly adults. *J Gerontol*. January 1987;42(1):82–85.

5. Goldstein J, Cajko L, Oosterbroek M, Michielsen M, van Houten O, Salverda F. Video games and the elderly. *Social Behavior and Personality*. 1997;25(4):345–52.

6. Torres A. Cognitive effects of videogames on older people. *Proc 7th ICDVRAT with ArtAbilitation*. 2008;191–98.

7. Basak C, Boot WR, Voss MW, Kramer AF. Can training in a real-time strategy video game attenuate cognitive decline in older adults? *Psychol Aging*. December 2008;23(4):765–77.

8. Stern Y, Blumen HM, Rich LW, Richards A, Herzberg G, Gopher D. Space Fortress game training and executive control in older adults: a pilot intervention. *Neuropsychol Dev Cogn B Aging Neuropsychol Cogn*. November 2011;18(6):653–77.

9. Loewenstein DA, Acevedo A, Czaja SJ, Duara R. Cognitive rehabilitation of mildly impaired Alzheimer disease patients on cholinesterase inhibitors. *Am J Geriatr Psychiatry*. July 2004;12(4):395–402.

10. Cipriani G, Bianchetti A, Trabucchi M. Outcomes of a computer-based cognitive rehabilitation program on Alzheimer's disease patients compared with those on patients affected by mild cognitive impairment. *Arch Gerontol Geriatr*. November 2006;43(3):327–35.

11. Tarraga L, Boada M, Modinos G, Espinosa A, Diego S, Morera A, Guitart M, Balcells J, Lopez OL, Becker JT. A randomised pilot study to assess the efficacy of an interactive, multimedia tool of cognitive stimulation in Alzheimer's disease. *J Neurol Neurosurg Psychiatry*. October 2006;77(10):1116–21.

12. Loewenstein et al. Cognitive rehabilitation of mildly impaired Alzheimer disease. *Am J Geriatr Psychiatry*.

13. Olazaran-Rodriguez J, Cruz-Orduna I, Jimenez-Martin F. Donepezil therapy in patients with vascular and post-traumatic cognitive impairment: some clinical observations. *Revista de Neurologia*. May 16, 2004;38(10):938–43.

14. Behrens TE, Johansen-Berg H, Woolrich MW, Smith SM, Wheeler-Kingshott CA, Boulby PA, Barker GJ, Sillery EL, Sheehan K, Ciccarelli O, Thompson AJ, Brady JM, Matthews PM. Non-invasive mapping of connections between human thalamus and cortex using diffusion imaging. *Nat Neurosci*. July 2003;6(7):750–57; Caeyenberghs K, Leemans A, Geurts M, Taymans T,

Vander LC, Smits-Engelsman BC, Sunaert S, Swinnen SP. Brain-behavior relationships in young traumatic brain injury patients: fractional anisotropy measures are highly correlated with dynamic visuomotor tracking performance. *Neuropsychologia*. April 2010;48(5):1472–82; Gold JJ, Smith CN, Bayley PJ, Shrager Y, Brewer JB, Stark CE, Hopkins RO, Squire LR. Item memory, source memory, and the medial temporal lobe: concordant findings from fMRI and memory-impaired patients. *Proc Natl Acad Sci USA*. June 13, 2006;103(24):9351–56; Voineskos AN, Rajji TK, Lobaugh NJ, Miranda D, Shenton ME, Kennedy JL, Pollock BG, Mulsant BH. Age-related decline in white matter tract integrity and cognitive performance: a DTI tractography and structural equation modeling study. *Neurobiol Aging*. April 1, 2010.

15. Becker JT, Mintun MA, Aleva K, Wiseman MB, Nichols T, DeKosky ST. Compensatory reallocation of brain resources supporting verbal episodic memory in Alzheimer's disease. *Neurology*. March 1996;46(3):692–700.

16. Dekosky ST, Scheff SW. Synapse loss in frontal cortex biopsies in Alzheimer's disease: correlation with cognitive severity. *Ann Neurol*. May 1990;27(5):457–64.

17. Tarraga et al. A randomised pilot study. *J Neurol Neurosurg Psychiatry*.

18. Sitzer DI, Twamley EW, Jeste DV. Cognitive training in Alzheimer's disease: a meta-analysis of the literature. *Acta Psychiatr Scand*. August 2006;114(2):75–90.

19. Cipriani et al. Outcomes of a computer-based cognitive rehabilitation program. *Arch Gerontol Geriatr*.

20. Farina E, Mantovani F, Fioravanti R, Pignatti R, Chiavari L, Imbornone E, Olivotto F, Alberoni M, Mariani C, Nemni R. Evaluating two group programmes of cognitive training in mild-to-moderate AD: is there any difference between a "global" stimulation and a "cognitive-specific" one? *Aging Ment Health*. May 2006;10(3):211–18.

21. Avila R, Bottino CM, Carvalho IA, Santos CB, Seral C, Miotto EC. Neuropsychological rehabilitation of memory deficits and activities of daily living in patients with Alzheimer's disease: a pilot study. *Braz J Med Biol Res*. November 2004;37(11):1721–29; Loewenstein et al. Cognitive rehabilitation of mildly impaired Alzheimer disease. *Am J Geriatr Psychiatry*.

22. Ibid.

23. Tippett WJ, Sergio LE. Visuomotor integration is impaired in early stage Alzheimer's disease. *Brain Res*. August 2, 2006;1102(1):92–102; Tippett WJ, Black SE. Regional cerebral blood flow correlates of visuospatial tasks in Alzheimer's disease. *J Int Neuropsychol Soc*. November 2008;14(6):1034–45.

24. Tippett, Sergio. Visuomotor integration is impaired. *Brain Res*; Tippett WJ, Krajewski A, Sergio LE. Visuomotor integration is compromised in Alzheimer's disease patients reaching for remembered targets. *Eur Neurol*.

2007;58(1):1–11; Tippett WJ, Sergio LE, Black SE. Compromised visually guided motor control in individuals with Alzheimer's disease: can reliable distinctions be observed? *J Clin Neurosci.* May 2012;19(5):655–60.

25. Knapp M, Thorgrimsen L, Patel A, Spector A, Hallam A, Woods B, Orrell M. Cognitive stimulation therapy for people with dementia: cost-effectiveness analysis. *Br J Psychiatry.* June 2006;188:574–80.

26. Ibid.

27. Zanetti O, Frisoni GB, De LD, Dello BM, Bianchetti A, Trabucchi M. Reality orientation therapy in Alzheimer disease: useful or not? A controlled study. *Alzheimer Dis Assoc Disord.* 1995;9(3):132–38.

28. Metitieri T, Zanetti O, Geroldi C, Frisoni GB, De LD, Dello BM, Bianchetti A, Trabucchi M. Reality orientation therapy to delay outcomes of progression in patients with dementia: a retrospective study. *Clin Rehabil.* October 2001;15(5):471–78; Orrell M, Spector A, Thorgrimsen L, Woods B. A pilot study examining the effectiveness of maintenance cognitive stimulation therapy (MCST) for people with dementia. *Int J Geriatr Psychiatry.* May 2005;20(5):446–51.

29. Bharwani G, Parikh PJ, Lawhorne LW, Van VE, Bharwani M. Individualized behavior management program for Alzheimer's/dementia residents using behavior-based ergonomic therapies. *Am J Alzheimers Dis Other Demen.* April 19, 2012.

30. Marcell J. If I only knew then—what I know now! Canadian Senior Years website. http://www.senioryears.com/ifionlyknew.html. Accessed January 19, 2013.

31. Our asks. Alzheimer's Society of Ontario website. http://championsfordementia.ca/our-asks/. Accessed January 19, 2013.

8. COGNITIVE ENHANCEMENTS

1. Lynch G, Palmer LC, Gall CM. The likelihood of cognitive enhancement. *Pharmacol Biochem Behav.* August 2011;99(2):116–29.

2. Lanni C, Lenzken SC, Pascale A, Del Vecchio, I, Racchi M, Pistoia F, Govoni S. Cognition enhancers between treating and doping the mind. *Pharmacol Res.* March 2008;57(3):199.

3. Partridge BJ, Bell SK, Lucke JC, Yeates S, Hall WD. Smart drugs "as common as coffee": media hype about neuroenhancement. *PLoS One.* 2011;6(11):e28416.

4. Lynch et al. The likelihood of cognitive enhancement. *Pharmacol Biochem Behav.*

5. Ibid.; Husain M, Mehta MA. Cognitive enhancement by drugs in health and disease. *Trends Cogn Sci.* January 2011;15(1):28–36.

6. Lynch et al. The likelihood of cognitive enhancement. *Pharmacol Biochem Behav.*

7. Lanni et al. Cognition enhancers. *Pharmacol Res.*

8. Herculano-Houzel S. The human brain in numbers: a linearly scaled-up primate brain. *Front Hum Neurosci* 2009;3:31.

9. WHAT IS MILD COGNITIVE IMPAIRMENT?

1. Mufson EJ, Binder L, Counts SE, Dekosky ST, de Toledo-Morrell L, Ginsberg SD, Ikonomovic MD, Perez SE, Scheff SW. Mild cognitive impairment: pathology and mechanisms. *Acta Neuropathol.* January 2012;123(1):13.

2. Braak H, Braak E. Staging of Alzheimer's disease-related neurofibrillary changes. *Neurobiol Aging.* May 1995;16(3):271–78.

3. Price JL, Morris JC. Tangles and plaques in nondemented aging and "preclinical" Alzheimer's disease. *Ann Neurol.* March 1999;45(3):358–68; Tippett WJ, Black SE. Regional cerebral blood flow correlates of visuospatial tasks in Alzheimer's disease. *J Int Neuropsychol Soc.* November 2008;14(6):1034–45.

4. Mufson et al. Mild cognitive impairment. *Acta Neuropathol.*

5. Nelson PT, Alafuzoff I, Bigio EH, Bouras C, Braak H, Cairns NJ, Castellani RJ, Crain BJ, Davies P, Tredici KD, Duyckaerts C, Frosch MP, Haroutunian V, Hof PR, Hulette CM, Hyman BT, Iwatsubo T, Jellinger KA, Jicha GA, Kovari E, Kukull WA, Leverenz JB, Love S, Mackenzie IR, Mann DM, Masliah E, McKee AC, Montine TJ, Morris JC, Schneider JA, Sonnen JA, Thal DR, Trojanowski JQ, Troncoso JC, Wisniewski T, Woltjer RL, Beach TG. Correlation of Alzheimer disease neuropathologic changes with cognitive status: a review of the literature. *J Neuropathol Exp Neurol.* May 2012;71(5):362–81.

6. Mufson et al. Mild cognitive impairment. *Acta Neuropathol*; Price JL, McKeel DW, Buckles VD, Roe CM, Xiong C, Grundman M, Hansen LA, Petersen RC, Parisi JE, Dickson DW, Smith CD, Davis DG, Schmitt FA, Markesbery WR, Kaye J, Kurlan R, Hulette C, Kurland BF, Higdon R, Kukull W, Morris JC. Neuropathology of nondemented aging: presumptive evidence for preclinical Alzheimer disease. *Neurobiol Aging.* July 2009;30(7):1026–36.

7. Hatanpaa K, Isaacs KR, Shirao T, Brady DR, Rapoport SI. Loss of proteins regulating synaptic plasticity in normal aging of the human brain and in Alzheimer disease. *J Neuropathol Exp Neurol.* June 1999;58(6):637–43; Hayashi K, Ishikawa R, Ye LH, He XL, Takata K, Kohama K, Shirao T. Mod-

ulatory role of drebrin on the cytoskeleton within dendritic spines in the rat cerebral cortex. *J Neurosci.* November 15, 1996;16(22):7161–70; Sultana R, Banks WA, Butterfield DA. Decreased levels of PSD95 and two associated proteins and increased levels of BCl2 and caspase 3 in hippocampus from subjects with amnestic mild cognitive impairment: insights into their potential roles for loss of synapses and memory, accumulation of Abeta, and neurode-generation in a prodromal stage of Alzheimer's disease. *J Neurosci Res.* February 15, 2010;88(3):469–77.

    8. Mufson et al. Mild cognitive impairment. *Acta Neuropathol.*

    9. Kendziorra K, Wolf H, Meyer PM, Barthel H, Hesse S, Becker GA, Luthardt J, Schildan A, Patt M, Sorger D, Seese A, Gertz HJ, Sabri O. De-creased cerebral alpha4beta2° nicotinic acetylcholine receptor availability in patients with mild cognitive impairment and Alzheimer's disease assessed with positron emission tomography. *Eur J Nucl Med Mol Imaging.* March 2011;38(3):515–25.

    10. Gabryelewicz T, Styczynska M, Luczywek E, Barczak A, Pfeffer A, An-drosiuk W, Chodakowska-Zebrowska M, Wasiak B, Peplonska B, Barcikowska M. The rate of conversion of mild cognitive impairment to dementia: predic-tive role of depression. *Int J Geriatr Psychiatry.* June 2007;22(6):563–67; Maioli F, Coveri M, Pagni P, Chiandetti C, Marchetti C, Ciarrocchi R, Rugge-ro C, Nativio V, Onesti A, D'Anastasio C, Pedone V. Conversion of mild cogni-tive impairment to dementia in elderly subjects: a preliminary study in a mem-ory and cognitive disorder unit. *Arch Gerontol Geriatr.* 2007;44(suppl 1):233–41.

    11. Hansson O, Zetterberg H, Buchhave P, Londos E, Blennow K, Minthon L. Association between CSF biomarkers and incipient Alzheimer's disease in patients with mild cognitive impairment: a follow-up study. *Lancet Neurol.* March 2006;5(3):228–34.

    12. Zhou B, Nakatani E, Teramukai S, Nagai Y, Fukushima M. Risk classifi-cation in mild cognitive impairment patients for developing Alzheimer's dis-ease. *J Alzheimers Dis.* March 16, 2012.

10. HOW DO I KNOW IF MY BRAIN IS AGING NORMALLY?

    1. Anstey KJ, Low LF. Normal cognitive changes in aging. *Aust Fam Phy-sician.* October 2004;33(10):783–87.

    2. Ibid.

    3. Wilson RS, Beckett LA, Barnes LL, Schneider JA, Bach J, Evans DA, Bennett DA. Individual differences in rates of change in cognitive abilities of older persons. *Psychol Aging.* June 2002;17(2):179–93.

4. Beason-Held LL, Kraut MA, Resnick SM. Longitudinal changes in aging brain function. *Neurobiol Aging.* April 2008;29(4):483–96.

5. Eyler LT, Sherzai A, Kaup AR, Jeste DV. A review of functional brain imaging correlates of successful cognitive aging. *Biol Psychiatry.* July 15, 2011;70(2):115–22.

6. Hagberg B, Bauer AB, Poon LW, Homma A. Cognitive functioning in centenarians: a coordinated analysis of results from three countries. *J Gerontol B Psychol Sci Soc Sci.* May 2001;56(3):141–51; Jeune B, Andersen-Ranberg K. [What can be learned from centenarians?] *Ugeskr Laeger.* November 15, 1999;161(46):6321–25; Ritchie K, Kildea D. Is senile dementia "age-related" or "ageing-related"?—evidence from meta-analysis of dementia prevalence in the oldest old. *Lancet.* October 7, 1995;346(8980):931–34.

7. Kliegel M, Moor C, Rott C. Cognitive status and development in the oldest old: a longitudinal analysis from the Heidelberg Centenarian Study. *Arch Gerontol Geriatr.* September 2004;39(2):143–56.

8. Ibid.; Anstey KJ, Luszcz MA, Giles LC, Andrews GR. Demographic, health, cognitive, and sensory variables as predictors of mortality in very old adults. *Psychol Aging.* March 2001;16(1):3–11.

9. Raz N, Gunning-Dixon FM, Head D, Dupuis JH, Acker JD. Neuroanatomical correlates of cognitive aging: evidence from structural magnetic resonance imaging. *Neuropsychology.* January 1998;12(1):95–114.

10. Ibid.

11. Ibid.

12. Schulte JN, Yarasheski KE. Effects of resistance training on the rate of muscle protein synthesis in frail elderly people. *Int J Sport Nutr Exerc Metab.* December 2001;11(suppl):S111–18.

13. Kwok V, Niu Z, Kay P, Zhou K, Mo L, Jin Z, So KF, Tan LH. Learning new color names produces rapid increase in gray matter in the intact adult human cortex. *Proc Natl Acad Sci USA.* April 19, 2011;108(16):6686–88.

14. Erickson KI, Voss MW, Prakash RS, Basak C, Szabo A, Chaddock L, Kim JS, Heo S, Alves H, White SM, Wojcicki TR, Mailey E, Vieira VJ, Martin SA, Pence BD, Woods JA, McAuley E, Kramer AF. Exercise training increases size of hippocampus and improves memory. *Proc Natl Acad Sci USA.* February 15, 2011;108(7):3017–22.

15. Zhou X, Merzenich MM. Developmentally degraded cortical temporal processing restored by training. *Nat Neurosci.* January 2009;12(1):26–28.

16. Good CD, Johnsrude IS, Ashburner J, Henson RN, Friston KJ, Frackowiak RS. A voxel-based morphometric study of ageing in 465 normal adult human brains. *Neuroimage.* July 2001;14(1):21–36.

17. Gautam P, Cherbuin N, Sachdev PS, Wen W, Anstey KJ. Relationships between cognitive function and frontal grey matter volumes and thickness in

middle aged and early old-aged adults: the PATH Through Life Study. *Neuro-image.* April 1, 2011;55(3):845–55.

18. Chantome M, Perruchet P, Hasboun D, Dormont D, Sahel M, Sourour N, Zouaoui A, Marsault C, Duyme M. Is there a negative correlation between explicit memory and hippocampal volume? *Neuroimage.* November 1999;10(5):589–95.

19. Bosch B, Bartres-Faz D, Rami L, Arenaza-Urquijo EM, Fernandez-Espejo D, Junque C, Sole-Padulles C, Sanchez-Valle R, Bargallo N, Falcon C, Molinuevo JL. Cognitive reserve modulates task-induced activations and deactivations in healthy elders, amnestic mild cognitive impairment and mild Alzheimer's disease. *Cortex.* April 2010;46(4):451–61; Stern Y, Habeck C, Moeller J, Scarmeas N, Anderson KE, Hilton HJ, Flynn J, Sackeim H, Van HR. Brain networks associated with cognitive reserve in healthy young and old adults. *Cereb Cortex.* April 2005;15(4):394–402.

20. Macdonald SW, Decarlo CA, Dixon RA. Linking biological and cognitive aging: toward improving characterizations of developmental time. *J Gerontol B Psychol Sci Soc Sci.* July 2011;66(suppl 1):i59–70.

21. Ibid.

22. Ibid.; Duthie SJ, Whalley LJ, Collins AR, Leaper S, Berger K, Deary IJ. Homocysteine, B vitamin status, and cognitive function in the elderly. *Am J Clin Nutr.* May 2002;75(5):908–13.

11. EXERCISE AND DIET

1. National Institutes of Health, U.S. Department of Health and Human Services, U.S Department of State, National Institute of Aging. Why population aging matters: a global perspective; 2007.

2. Lind J. *A Treatise of the Scurvy.* Edinburgh: A. Millar; 1753.

3. Statistics Canada. Canadian community health survey, nurition; 2004.

4. Garry PJ, VanderJagt DJ, Hunt WC. Ascorbic acid intakes and plasma levels in healthy elderly. *Ann NY Acad Sci.* 1987;498:90–99.

5. Dorjgochoo T, Deming SL, Gao YT, Lu W, Zheng Y, Ruan Z, Zheng W, Shu XO. History of benign breast disease and risk of breast cancer among women in China: a case-control study. *Cancer Causes Control.* October 2008;19(8):819–28.

6. Fotherby MD, Williams JC, Forster LA, Craner P, Ferns GA. Effect of vitamin C on ambulatory blood pressure and plasma lipids in older persons. *J Hypertens.* April 2000;18(4):411–15.

7. Harrison FE, May JM. Vitamin C function in the brain: vital role of the ascorbate transporter SVCT2. *Free Radic Biol Med.* March 15, 2009;46(6):719–30.

8. Ibid.

9. Institute of Medicine, Food and Nutrition Board. *Dietary Reference Intakes for Vitamin A, Vitamin K, Arsenic, Boron, Chromium, Copper, Iodine, Iron, Manganese, Molybdenum, Nickel, Silicon, Vanadium and Zinic.* Washington, DC: National Academy Press; 2001.

10. Zeba AN, Sorgho H, Rouamba N, Zongo I, Rouamba J, Guiguemde RT, Hamer DH, Mokhtar N, Ouedraogo JB. Major reduction of malaria morbidity with combined vitamin A and zinc supplementation in young children in Burkina Faso: a randomized double blind trial. *Nutr J.* 2008;7:7.

11. Institute of Medicine. *Dietary Reference Intakes for Vitamin A*

12. Masterjohn C. Vitamin D toxicity redefined: vitamin K and the molecular mechanism. *Med Hypotheses.* 2007;68(5):1026–34.

13. Fillenbaum GG, Kuchibhatla MN, Hanlon JT, Artz MB, Pieper CF, Schmader KE, Dysken MW, Gray SL. Dementia and Alzheimer's disease in community-dwelling elders taking vitamin C and/or vitamin E. *Ann Pharmacother.* December 2005;39(12):2009–14; Landmark K. [Could intake of vitamins C and E inhibit development of Alzheimer dementia?] *Tidsskr Nor Laegeforen.* January 12, 2006;126(2):159–61.

14. Buell JS, Dawson-Hughes B. Vitamin D and neurocognitive dysfunction: preventing "D"ecline? *Mol Aspects Med.* December 2008;29(6):415–22; Zittermann A, Schleithoff SS, Koerfer R. Markers of bone metabolism in congestive heart failure. *Clin Chim Acta.* April 2006;366(1–2):27–36.

15. Zittermann A, Schleithoff SS, Koerfer R. Putting cardiovascular disease and vitamin D insufficiency into perspective. *Br J Nutr.* October 2005;94(4):483–92.

16. Annweiler C, Schott AM, Rolland Y, Blain H, Herrmann FR, Beauchet O. Dietary intake of vitamin D and cognition in older women: a large population-based study. *Neurology.* November 16, 2010;75(20):1810–86.

17. Annweiler C, Schott AM, Berrut G, Fantino B, Beauchet O. Vitamin D-related changes in physical performance: a systematic review. *J Nutr Health Aging.* December 2009;13(10):893–98.

18. Azzi A, Stocker A. Vitamin E: non-antioxidant roles. *Prog Lipid Res.* May 2000;39(3):231–55; Schneider C. Chemistry and biology of vitamin E. *Mol Nutr Food Res.* January 2005;49(1):7–30; Villacorta L, Graca-Souza AV, Ricciarelli R, Zingg JM, Azzi A. Alpha-tocopherol induces expression of connective tissue growth factor and antagonizes tumor necrosis factor-alpha-mediated downregulation in human smooth muscle cells. *Circ Res.* January 10, 2003;92(1):104–10.

19. Muller DP. Vitamin E and neurological function. *Mol Nutr Food Res.* May 2010;54(5):710–18.

20. Brigelius-Flohe R. Vitamin E: the shrew waiting to be tamed. *Free Radic Biol Med.* March 1, 2009;46(5):543–54.

21. Ames D, Ritchie C. Antioxidants and Alzheimer's disease: time to stop feeding vitamin E to dementia patients? *Int Psychogeriatr.* February 2007;19(1):1–8.

22. Petersen RC, Thomas RG, Grundman M, Bennett D, Doody R, Ferris S, Galasko D, Jin S, Kaye J, Levey A, Pfeiffer E, Sano M, van Dyck CH, Thal LJ. Vitamin E and donepezil for the treatment of mild cognitive impairment. *N Engl J Med.* June 9, 2005;352(23):2379–88.

23. Miller ER, Pastor-Barriuso R, Dalal D, Riemersma RA, Appel LJ, Guallar E. Meta-analysis: high dosage vitamin E supplementation may increase all-cause mortality. *Ann Int Med.* 2005;142:37–46.

24. Sun AY, Simonyi A, Sun GY (2002) The "French Paradox" and beyond: neuroprotective effects of polyphenols. Free Radic Biol Med 32:314-318

25. Sun AY, Simonyi A, Sun GY (2002) The "French Paradox" and beyond: neuroprotective effects of polyphenols. Free Radic Biol Med 32:314-318

26. Neves R, Lucio A, Lima LC, Reis S (2012) Resveratrol in Medicinal Chemistry: A Critical Review of its Pharmacokinetics, Drug-Delivery, and Membrane Interactions. Bentham Science Publishers, pp 1663-1681

27. Walle T, Hsieh F, DeLegge MH, Oatis JE, Walle UK. High absorption but very low bioavailability of oral resveratrol in humans. *Drug Metab Dispos.* December 2004;32(12):1377–82.

28. Richard T, Pawlus AD, Iglesias ML, Pedrot E, Waffo-Teguo P, Merillon JM, Monti JP. Neuroprotective properties of resveratrol and derivatives. *Ann NY Acad Sci.* January 2011;1215:103–8.

29. Ibid.; Albani D, Polito L, Signorini A, Forloni G. Neuroprotective properties of resveratrol in different neurodegenerative disorders. *Biofactors.* September 2010;36(5):370–76.

30. Huber K, Superti-Furga G. After the grape rush: sirtuins as epigenetic drug targets in neurodegenerative disorders. *Bioorg Med Chem.* January 15, 2011.

31. Mattson MP. Neuroprotective signaling and the aging brain: take away my food and let me run. *Brain Res.* December 15, 2000;886(1–2):47–53.

32. Lane MA, Ingram DK, Ball SS, Roth GS. Dehydroepiandrosterone sulfate: a biomarker of primate aging slowed by calorie restriction. *J Clin Endocrinol Metab.* July 1997;82(7):2093–96; Roth GS, Lesnikov V, Lesnikov M, Ingram DK, Lane MA. Dietary caloric restriction prevents the age-related decline in plasma melatonin levels of rhesus monkeys. *J Clin Endocrinol Metab.* July 2001;86(7):3292–95; Ingram DK, Cutler RG, Weindruch R, Ren-

quist DM, Knapka JJ, April M, Belcher CT, Clark MA, Hatcherson CD, Marriott BM. Dietary restriction and aging: the initiation of a primate study. *J Gerontol.* September 1990;45(5):B148–63.

33. Mattson. Neuroprotective signaling and the aging brain. *Brain Res*; Fratiglioni L, Mangialasche F, Qiu C. Brain aging: lessons from community studies. *Nutr Rev.* December 2010;68(suppl 2):S119–27; Haan MN, Wallace R. Can dementia be prevented? Brain aging in a population-based context. *Annu Rev Public Health.* 2004;25:1–24.

34. Friedman R, Tappen RM. The effect of planned walking on communication in Alzheimer's disease. *J Am Geriatr Soc.* July 1991;39(7):650–54.

35. Scherder EJ, Van PJ, Deijen JB, Van Der KS, Orlebeke JF, Burgers I, Devriese PP, Swaab DF, Sergeant JA. Physical activity and executive functions in the elderly with mild cognitive impairment. *Aging Ment Health.* May 2005;9(3):272–80.

36. Sobel BP. Bingo vs. physical intervention in stimulating short-term cognition in Alzheimer's disease patients. *Am J Alzheimers Dis Other Demen.* March 2001;16(2):115–20.

37. Rolland Y, Rival L, Pillard F, Lafont C, Rivere D, Albarede J, Vellas B. Feasibility of regular physical exercise for patients with moderate to severe Alzheimer disease. *J Nutr Health Aging.* 2000;4(2):109–13.

38. Abbott RD, White LR, Ross GW, Masaki KH, Curb JD, Petrovitch H. Walking and dementia in physically capable elderly men. *JAMA.* September 22, 2004;292(12):1447–53.

39. Larson EB, Wang L, Bowen JD, McCormick WC, Teri L, Crane P, Kukull W. Exercise is associated with reduced risk for incident dementia among persons 65 years of age and older. *Ann Intern Med.* January 17, 2006;144(2):73–81.

40. Pereira AC, Huddleston DE, Brickman AM, Sosunov AA, Hen R, McKhann GM, Sloan R, Gage FH, Brown TR, Small SA. An in vivo correlate of exercise-induced neurogenesis in the adult dentate gyrus. *Proc Natl Acad Sci USA.* March 27, 2007;104(13):5638–43.

41. Nichol KE, Parachikova AI, Cotman CW. Three weeks of running wheel exposure improves cognitive performance in the aged Tg2576 mouse. *Behav Brain Res.* December 3, 2007;184(2):124–32.

42. Van Gelder BM, Tijhuis MA, Kalmijn S, Giampaoli S, Nissinen A, Kromhout D. Physical activity in relation to cognitive decline in elderly men: the FINE Study. *Neurology.* December 28, 2004;63(12):2316–21; Verghese J, Lipton RB, Katz MJ, Hall CB, Derby CA, Kuslansky G, Ambrose AF, Sliwinski M, Buschke H. Leisure activities and the risk of dementia in the elderly. *N Engl J Med.* June 19, 2003;348(25):2508–16.

12. HEAD AND HEART, THE CONNECTION WE SHOULD NEVER FORGET!

1. Gorelick PB, Scuteri A, Black SE, Decarli C, Greenberg SM, Iadecola C, Launer LJ, Laurent S, Lopez OL, Nyenhuis D, Petersen RC, Schneider JA, Tzourio C, Arnett DK, Bennett DA, Chui HC, Higashida RT, Lindquist R, Nilsson PM, Roman GC, Sellke FW, Seshadri S. Vascular contributions to cognitive impairment and dementia: a statement for healthcare professionals from the American Heart Association/American Stroke Association. *Stroke.* September 2011;42(9):2672–2713; Saposnik G, Cote R, Rochon PA, Mamdani M, Liu Y, Raptis S, Kapral MK, Black SE. Care and outcomes in patients with ischemic stroke with and without preexisting dementia. *Neurology.* November 1, 2011;77(18):1664–73.

2. Gorelick et al. Vascular contributions to cognitive impairment. *Stroke.*

3. Moreau F, Jeerakathil T, Coutts SB, FRCPC for the ASPIRE investigators. Patients referred for TIA may still have persisting neurological deficits. *Can J Neurol Sci.* March 2012;39(2):170–73.

4. Pettersen JA, Sathiyamoorthy G, Gao FQ, Szilagyi G, Nadkarni NK, St George-Hyslop P, Rogaeva E, Black SE. Microbleed topography, leukoaraiosis, and cognition in probable Alzheimer disease from the Sunnybrook dementia study. *Arch Neurol.* June 2008;65(6):790–95.

5. Gorelick et al. Vascular contributions to cognitive impairment. *Stroke.*

6. Ibid.

7. Ibid.

8. Ibid.

9. Ibid.

10. Ibid.; Hachinski VC, Lassen NA, Marshall J. Multi-infarct dementia: a cause of mental deterioration in the elderly. *Lancet.* July 27, 1974;2(7874):207–10; Tomlinson BE, Blessed G, Roth M. Observations on the brains of demented old people. *J Neurol Sci.* September 1970;11(3):205–42.

11. Madureira S, Canhao P, Guerreiro M, Ferro JM. Cognitive and emotional consequences of perimesencephalic subarachnoid hemorrhage. *J Neurol.* November 2000;247(11):862–67; Pendlebury ST, Rothwell PM. Prevalence, incidence, and factors associated with pre-stroke and post-stroke dementia: a systematic review and meta-analysis. *Lancet Neurol.* November 2009;8(11):1006–18.

12. Pendlebury, Rothwell. Prevalence, incidence, and factors associated with pre-stroke and post-stroke dementia. *Lancet Neurol.*; Pendlebury ST. Stroke-related dementia: rates, risk factors and implications for future research. *Maturitas.* November 20, 2009;64(3):165–71.

13. Madureira et al. Cognitive and emotional consequences of perimesen-cephalic subarachnoid hemorrhage. *J Neurol.*

14. Ibid.

15. Reitz C, Bos MJ, Hofman A, Koudstaal PJ, Breteler MM. Prestroke cognitive performance, incident stroke, and risk of dementia: the Rotterdam Study. *Stroke.* January 2008;39(1):36–41.

16. Pendlebury ST, Rothwell PM. Risk of recurrent stroke, other vascular events and dementia after transient ischaemic attack and stroke. *Cerebrovasc Dis.* 2009;27(suppl 3):1–11.

17. Pendlebury ST, Wadling S, Silver LE, Mehta Z, Rothwell PM. Transient cognitive impairment in TIA and minor stroke. *Stroke.* November 2011;42(11):3116–21.

18. Ibid.

19. Ibid.

20. Jacquin A, Aboa-Eboule C, Rouaud O, Osseby GV, Binquet C, Durier J, Moreau T, Bonithon-Kopp C, Giroud M, Bejot Y. Prior transient ischemic attack and dementia after subsequent ischemic stroke. *Alzheimer Dis Assoc Disord.* December 20, 2011.

21. Gorelick et al. Vascular contributions to cognitive impairment. *Stroke.*

22. Howard G, Wagenknecht LE, Cai J, Cooper L, Kraut MA, Toole JF. Cigarette smoking and other risk factors for silent cerebral infarction in the general population. *Stroke.* May 1998;29(5):913–17; Price TR, Manolio TA, Kronmal RA, Kittner SJ, Yue NC, Robbins J, Anton-Culver H, O'Leary DH. Silent brain infarction on magnetic resonance imaging and neurological abnor-malities in community-dwelling older adults: the Cardiovascular Health Study, CHS Collaborative Research Group. *Stroke.* June 1997;28(6):1158–64; Verm-eer SE, Koudstaal PJ, Oudkerk M, Hofman A, Breteler MM. Prevalence and risk factors of silent brain infarcts in the population-based Rotterdam Scan Study. *Stroke.* January 2002;33(1):21–25; Vermeer SE, den HT, Koudstaal PJ, Oudkerk M, Hofman A, Breteler MM. Incidence and risk factors of silent brain infarcts in the population-based Rotterdam Scan Study. *Stroke.* February 2003;34(2):392–96.

23. Vermeer et al. Incidence and risk factors of silent brain infarcts. *Stroke.*

24. Ibid.

25. Hoffmann T, Bennett S, Koh CL, McKenna K. A systematic review of cognitive interventions to improve functional ability in people who have cognitive impairment following stroke. *Top Stroke Rehabil.* March 2010;17(2):99–107.

26. Ibid.

27. Hockey R, Gaillard AWK, Coles MGH, North Atlantic Treaty Organization, Scientific Affairs Division. *Energetics and Human Information Process-*

ing. Dordrecht: Nijhoff; 1986; Lambourne K, Tomporowski P. The effect of exercise-induced arousal on cognitive task performance: a meta-regression analysis. *Brain Res.* June 23, 2010;1341:12–24; Tomporowski PD. Effects of acute bouts of exercise on cognition. *Acta Psychol (Amst).* March 2003;112(3):297–324.

28. Lambourne, Tomporowski. The effect of exercise-induced arousal on cognitive task performance. *Brain Res.*

29. McMorris T, Omporowski P, Audiffren M. *Exercise and Cognitive Function.* Chichester, UK: Wiley-Blackwell; 2009.

30. Ibid.

31. Angevaren M, Aufdemkampe G, Verhaar HJ, Aleman A, Vanhees L. Physical activity and enhanced fitness to improve cognitive function in older people without known cognitive impairment. *Cochrane Database Syst Rev.* 2008;(3):CD005381.

32. Go to www.heartandstroke.com for more information on these symptoms.

33. The FAST acronym is taken from http://www.cpmc.org/advanced/neurosciences/stroke/patients/fast.html.

13. NEUROPLASTICITY AND COGNITIVE PLASTICITY

1. Jernigan TL, Archibald SL, Fennema-Notestine C, Gamst AC, Stout JC, Bonner J, Hesselink JR. Effects of age on tissues and regions of the cerebrum and cerebellum. *Neurobiol Aging.* July 2001;22(4):581–94.

2. Van PC. Relationship between hippocampal volume and memory ability in healthy individuals across the lifespan: review and meta-analysis. *Neuropsychologia.* 2004;42(10):1394–1413; Van PC, Plante E, Davidson PS, Kuo TY, Bajuscak L, Glisky EL. Memory and executive function in older adults: relationships with temporal and prefrontal gray matter volumes and white matter hyperintensities. *Neuropsychologia.* 2004;42(10):1313–35.

3. Gunning-Dixon FM, Raz N. The cognitive correlates of white matter abnormalities in normal aging: a quantitative review. *Neuropsychology.* April 2000;14(2):224–32; Raz N, Williamson A, Gunning-Dixon F, Head D, Acker JD. Neuroanatomical and cognitive correlates of adult age differences in acquisition of a perceptual-motor skill. *Microsc Res Tech.* October 1, 2000;51(1):85–93.

4. Bartzokis G, Beckson M, Lu PH, Nuechterlein KH, Edwards N, Mintz J. Age-related changes in frontal and temporal lobe volumes in men: a magnetic resonance imaging study. *Arch Gen Psychiatry.* May 2001;58(5):461–65.

5. Van et al. Memory and executive function in older adults. *Neuropsychologia*; Rodrigue KM, Raz N. Shrinkage of the entorhinal cortex over five years predicts memory performance in healthy adults. *J Neurosci.* January 28, 2004;24(4):956–63.

6. Burggren AC, Renner B, Jones M, Donix M, Suthana NA, Martin-Harris L, Ercoli LM, Miller KJ, Siddarth P, Small GW, Bookheimer SY. Thickness in entorhinal and subicular cortex predicts episodic memory decline in mild cognitive impairment. *Int J Alzheimers Dis.* 2011;2011:956053; Catenoix H, Magnin M, Mauguiere F, Ryvlin P. Evoked potential study of hippocampal efferent projections in the human brain. *Clin Neurophysiol.* June 11, 2011; Stranahan AM, Salas-Vega S, Jiam NT, Gallagher M. Interference with reelin signaling in the lateral entorhinal cortex impairs spatial memory. *Neurobiol Learn Mem.* September 2011;96(2):150–55.

7. Wingfield A, Grossman M. Language and the aging brain: patterns of neural compensation revealed by functional brain imaging. *J Neurophysiol.* December 2006;96(6):2830–39; Greenwood PM, Parasuraman R. Neuronal and cognitive plasticity: a neurocognitive framework for ameliorating cognitive aging. *Front Aging Neurosci.* 2010;2:150.

8. Cabeza R, Anderson ND, Locantore JK, McIntosh AR. Aging gracefully: compensatory brain activity in high-performing older adults. *Neuroimage.* November 2002;17(3):1394–1402; Persson J, Nyberg L. Altered brain activity in healthy seniors: what does it mean? *Prog Brain Res.* 2006;157:45–56.

9. Persson, Nyberg. Altered brain activity in healthy seniors. *Prog Brain Res.*

10. Ibid.; Cabeza R. Cognitive neuroscience of aging: contributions of functional neuroimaging. *Scand J Psychol.* July 2001;42(3):277–86.

11. Cabeza. Cognitive neuroscience of aging. *Scand J Psychol.*

12. Carlson NR. *Physiology of Behavior*. 10 ed. Boston: Allyn & Bacon; 2010.

13. Giedd JN. Structural magnetic resonance imaging of the adolescent brain. *Ann NY Acad Sci.* June 2004;1021:77–85.

14. Weiss B. Can endocrine disruptors influence neuroplasticity in the aging brain? *Neurotoxicology.* September 2007;28(5):938–50.

15. Deng W, Aimone JB, Gage FH. New neurons and new memories: how does adult hippocampal neurogenesis affect learning and memory? *Nat Rev Neurosci.* May 2010;11(5):339–50.

16. Ibid.

17. Weiss B. Can endocrine disruptors influence neuroplasticity in the aging brain? *Neurotoxicology.*

18. Ramirez-Amaya V, Marrone DF, Gage FH, Worley PF, Barnes CA. Integration of new neurons into functional neural networks. *J Neurosci.* November 22, 2006;26(47):12237–41.

19. Weiss B. Can endocrine disruptors influence neuroplasticity in the aging brain? *Neurotoxicology.*

20. Van Kampen JM, Robertson HA. A possible role for dopamine D3 receptor stimulation in the induction of neurogenesis in the adult rat substantia nigra. *Neuroscience.* 2005;136(2):381–86.

21. Park DC, Reuter-Lorenz P. The adaptive brain: aging and neurocognitive scaffolding. *Annu Rev Psychol.* 2009;60:173–96.

22. Ibid.

23. Davis SW, Dennis NA, Daselaar SM, Fleck MS, Cabeza R. Que PASA? The posterior-anterior shift in aging. *Cereb Cortex.* May 2008;18(5):1201–9.

24. Reuter-Lorenz PA, Lustig C. Brain aging: reorganizing discoveries about the aging mind. *Curr Opin Neurobiol.* April 2005;15(2):245–51.

25. Park, Reuter-Lorenz. The adaptive brain. *Annu Rev Psychol.*

26. Patients with locked-in syndrome will soon be able to communicate with mind-reading technology, predicts scientist. *Daily Mail.* September 21, 2010.

27. Ibid.

28. Owen AM, Coleman MR. Using neuroimaging to detect awareness in disorders of consciousness. *Funct Neurol.* October 2008;23(4):189–94.

29. Patients with locked-in syndrome. *Daily Mail.*

30. Lowdon P, Murray A, Langley P. Heart rate and blood pressure interactions during attempts to consciously raise or lower heart rate and blood pressure in normotensive subjects. *Physiol Meas.* March 2011;32(3):359–67.

31. Long J, Li Y, Wang H, Yu T, Pan J, Li F. A hybrid brain computer interface to control the direction and speed of a simulated or real wheelchair. *IEEE Trans Neural Syst Rehabil Eng.* September 2012;20(5):720–29.

32. Cincotti F, Aloise F, Bufalari S, Schalk G, Oriolo G, Cherubini A, Davide F, Babiloni F, Marciani MG, Mattia D. Non-invasive brain-computer interface system to operate assistive devices. *Conf Proc IEEE Eng Med Biol Soc.* 2007;2007:2532–35; Vaughan TM, McFarland DJ, Schalk G, Sarnacki WA, Krusienski DJ, Sellers EW, Wolpaw JR. The Wadsworth BCI Research and Development Program: at home with BCI. *IEEE Trans Neural Syst Rehabil Eng.* June 2006;14(2):229–33.

33. Hochberg LR, Serruya MD, Friehs GM, Mukand JA, Saleh M, Caplan AH, Branner A, Chen D, Penn RD, Donoghue JP. Neuronal ensemble control of prosthetic devices by a human with tetraplegia. *Nature.* July 13, 2006;442(7099):164–71.

34. The company's website at www.emotiv.com provides more information.

35. Encinas JM, Michurina TV, Peunova N, Park JH, Tordo J, Peterson DA, Fishell G, Koulakov A, Enikolopov G. Division-coupled astrocytic differentiation and age-related depletion of neural stem cells in the adult hippocampus. *Cell Stem Cell.* May 6, 2011;8(5):566–79.

36. Chojnacki AK, Mak GK, Weiss S. Identity crisis for adult periventricular neural stem cells: subventricular zone astrocytes, ependymal cells or both? *Nat Rev Neurosci.* February 2009;10(2):153–63; Kolb B, Morshead C, Gonzalez C, Kim M, Gregg C, Shingo T, Weiss S. Growth factor-stimulated generation of new cortical tissue and functional recovery after stroke damage to the motor cortex of rats. *J Cereb Blood Flow Metab.* May 2007;27(5):983–97.

37. Yoshikawa G, Momiyama T, Oya S, Takai K, Tanaka J, Higashiyama S, Saito N, Kirino T, Kawahara N. Induction of striatal neurogenesis and generation of region-specific functional mature neurons after ischemia by growth factors: laboratory investigation. *J Neurosurg.* October 2010;113(4):835–50.

38. Rando TA. Stem cells, ageing and the quest for immortality. *Nature.* June 29, 2006;441(7097):1080–86.

39. Rando TA, Chang HY. Aging, rejuvenation, and epigenetic reprogramming: resetting the aging clock. *Cell.* January 20, 2012;148(1–2):46–57.

40. Siren AL, Radyushkin K, Boretius S, Kammer D, Riechers CC, Natt O, Sargin D, Watanabe T, Sperling S, Michaelis T, Price J, Meyer B, Frahm J, Ehrenreich H. Global brain atrophy after unilateral parietal lesion and its prevention by erythropoietin. *Brain.* February 2006;129(2):480–89.

41. Berger TW, Hampson RE, Song D, Goonawardena A, Marmarelis VZ, Deadwyler SA. A cortical neural prosthesis for restoring and enhancing memory. *J Neural Eng.* August 2011;8(4):046017.

42. Kurzweil R. Human life: the next generation. *New Scientist.* September 24, 2005.

43. Kindratenko V. Trends in high-performance computing. *Computing Sci Eng.* May 2011;13(3):92–95.

44. Kurzweil. Human life. *New Scientist.*

45. Ibid.; Voelbel GT, Genova HM, Chiaravalotti ND, Hoptman MJ. Diffusion tensor imaging of traumatic brain injury review: implications for neurorehabilitation. *NeuroRehabilitation.* January 1, 2012;31(3):281–93.

46. Kurzweil. Human life. *New Scientist.*

47. Markram H. The blue brain project. *Nat Rev Neurosci.* February 2006;7(2):153–60.

48. Feldman M. The next step in human brain simulation. *HPC Wire.* July 11, 2011.

REFERENCES

Abbott RD, White LR, Ross GW, Masaki KH, Curb JD, and Petrovitch H. 2004. Walking and dementia in physically capable elderly men. *JAMA* 292 (12): 1447–53.

Albani D, Polito L, Signorini A, and Forloni G. 2010. Neuroprotective properties of resveratrol in different neurodegenerative disorders. *Biofactors* 36 (5): 370–76.

Alkire MT, Haier RJ, Fallon JH, and Cahill L. 1998. Hippocampal, but not amygdala, activity at encoding correlates with long-term, free recall of nonemotional information. *Proc Natl Acad Sci USA* 95 (24): 14506–10.

Alzheimer's Society Canada. 2013. http://www.alzheimer.ca/en/Living-with-dementia/Treatment-options/Drugs-approved-for-Alzheimers-disease.

Alzheimer's Society U.K. 2013. http://www.alzheimers.org.uk/site/scripts documents_info.php?documentID=147.

Alzheimer's Society U.S. 2013. http://www.alz.org/research/science/alzheimers_disease_treatments.asp#approved.

Ames D, and Ritchie C. 2007. Antioxidants and Alzheimer's disease: time to stop feeding vitamin E to dementia patients? *Int Psychogeriatr* 19 (1): 1–8.

Angevaren M, Aufdemkampe G, Verhaar HJ, Aleman A, and Vanhees L. 2008. Physical activity and enhanced fitness to improve cognitive function in older people without known cognitive impairment. *Cochrane Database Syst Rev* (3): CD005381.

Annweiler C, Schott AM, Berrut G, Fantino B, and Beauchet O. 2009. Vitamin D-related changes in physical performance: a systematic review. *J Nutr Health Aging* 13 (10): 893–98.

Annweiler C, Schott AM, Rolland Y, Blain H, Herrmann FR, and Beauchet O. 2010. Dietary intake of vitamin D and cognition in older women: a large population-based study. *Neurology* 75 (20): 1810–16.

Anstey KJ, and Low LF. 2004. Normal cognitive changes in aging. *Aust Fam Physician* 33 (10): 783–87.

Anstey KJ, Luszcz MA, Giles LC, and Andrews GR. 2001. Demographic, health, cognitive, and sensory variables as predictors of mortality in very old adults. *Psychol Aging* 16 (1): 3–11.

Avila R, Bottino CM, Carvalho IA, Santos CB, Seral C, and Miotto EC. 2004. Neuropsychological rehabilitation of memory deficits and activities of daily living in patients with Alzheimer's disease: a pilot study. *Braz J Med Biol Res* 37 (11): 1721–29.

Azzi A, and Stocker A. 2000. Vitamin E: non-antioxidant roles. *Prog Lipid Res* 39 (3): 231–55.

Bartzokis G, Beckson M, Lu PH, Nuechterlein KH, Edwards N, and Mintz J. 2001. Age-related changes in frontal and temporal lobe volumes in men: a magnetic resonance imaging study. *Arch Gen Psychiatry* 58 (5): 461–65.

Bartzokis G, Cummings JL, Sultzer D, Henderson VW, Nuechterlein KH, and Mintz J. 2003. White matter structural integrity in healthy aging adults and patients with Alzheimer disease: a magnetic resonance imaging study. *Arch Neurol* 60 (3): 393–98.

Basak C, Boot WR, Voss MW, and Kramer AF. 2008. Can training in a real-time strategy video game attenuate cognitive decline in older adults? *Psychol Aging* 23 (4): 765–77.

Bayles KA, and Tomoeda CK. 1991. Caregiver report of prevalence and appearance order of linguistic symptoms in Alzheimer's patients. *Gerontologist* 31 (2): 210–16.

Beason-Held LL, Kraut MA, and Resnick SM. 2008. Longitudinal changes in aging brain function. *Neurobiol Aging* 29 (4): 483–96.

Becker JT, Mintun MA, Aleva K, Wiseman MB, Nichols T, and DeKosky ST. 1996. Compensatory reallocation of brain resources supporting verbal episodic memory in Alzheimer's disease. *Neurology* 46 (3): 692–700.

Behrens TE, Johansen-Berg H, Woolrich MW, Smith SM, Wheeler-Kingshott CA, Boulby PA, Barker GJ, Sillery EL, Sheehan K, Ciccarelli O, Thompson AJ, Brady JM, and Matthews PM. 2003. Non-invasive mapping of connections between human thalamus and cortex using diffusion imaging. *Nat Neurosci* 6 (7): 750–57.

Benton AL. 1994. Neuropsychological assessment. *Annual Review of Psychology* 45:1–23.

Berger TW, Hampson RE, Song D, Goonawardena A, Marmarelis VZ, and Deadwyler SA. 2011. A cortical neural prosthesis for restoring and enhancing memory. *J Neural Eng* 8 (4): 046017.

Bharwani G, Parikh PJ, Lawhorne LW, Van VE, and Bharwani M. 2012. Individualized behavior management program for Alzheimer's/dementia residents using behavior-based ergonomic therapies. *Am J Alzheimers Dis Other Demen* 27 (3):188–95.

Bialystok E, and Craik FI. 2007. Bilingualism and naming: implications for cognitive assessment. *J Int Neuropsychol Soc.* 13 (2): 209–11.

Binder JR, Gross WL, Allendorfer JB, Bonilha L, Chapin J, Edwards JC, Grabowski TJ, Langfitt JT, Loring DW, Lowe MJ, Koenig K, Morgan PS, Ojemann JG, Rorden C, Szaflarski JP, Tivarus ME, and Weaver KE. 2011. Mapping anterior temporal lobe language areas with fMRI: a multicenter normative study. *Neuroimage* 54 (2): 1465–75.

Blennow K, de Leon MJ, and Zetterberg H. 2006. Alzheimer's disease. *Lancet* 368 (9533): 387–403.

Bookheimer SY, Zeffiro IA, Blaxton T, Gaillard W, and Theodore W. 1995. Regional cerebral blood flow during object naming and word reading. *Human Brain Mapping* 3 (2): 93–106.

Boot WR, Kramer AF, Simons DJ, Fabiani M, and Gratton G. 2008. The effects of video game playing on attention, memory, and executive control. *Acta Psychol (Amst)* 129 (3): 387–98.

Bosch B, Bartres-Faz D, Rami L, Arenaza-Urquijo EM, Fernandez-Espejo D, Junque C, Sole-Padulles C, Sanchez-Valle R, Bargallo N, Falcon C, and Molinuevo JL. 2010. Cognitive reserve modulates task-induced activations and deactivations in healthy elders, amnestic mild cognitive impairment and mild Alzheimer's disease. *Cortex* 46 (4): 451–61.

Bowles KH, and Baugh AC. 2007. Applying research evidence to optimize telehomecare. *J Cardiovasc Nurs* 22 (1): 5–15.

Bozeat S, Gregory CA, Ralph MA, and Hodges JR. 2000. Which neuropsychiatric and behavioural features distinguish frontal and temporal variants of frontotemporal dementia from Alzheimer's disease? *J Neurol Neurosurg Psychiatry* 69 (2): 178–86.

Braak H, and Braak E. 1995. Staging of Alzheimer's disease-related neurofibrillary changes. *Neurobiol Aging* 16 (3): 271–78.

Brigelius-Flohe R. 2009. Vitamin E: the shrew waiting to be tamed. *Free Radic Biol Med* 46 (5): 543–54.

Buell JS, and Dawson-Hughes B. 2008. Vitamin D and neurocognitive dysfunction: preventing "D"ecline? *Mol Aspects Med* 29 (6): 415–22.

Burggren AC, Renner B, Jones M, Donix M, Suthana NA, Martin-Harris L, Ercoli LM, Miller KJ, Siddarth P, Small GW, and Bookheimer SY. 2011. Thickness in entorhinal and subicular cortex predicts episodic memory decline in mild cognitive impairment. *Int J Alzheimers Dis*: 956053.

Cabeza R. 2001. Cognitive neuroscience of aging: contributions of functional neuroimaging. *Scand J Psychol* 42 (3): 277–86.

Cabeza R. 2002. Hemispheric asymmetry reduction in older adults: the HAROLD model. *Psychol Aging* 17 (1): 85–100.

Cabeza R, Anderson ND, Locantore JK, and McIntosh AR. 2002. Aging gracefully: compensatory brain activity in high-performing older adults. *Neuroimage* 17 (3): 1394–1402.

Caeyenberghs K, Leemans A, Geurts M, Taymans T, Vander LC, Smits-Engelsman BC, Sunaert S, and Swinnen SP. 2010. Brain-behavior relationships in young traumatic brain injury patients: fractional anisotropy measures are highly correlated with dynamic visuomotor tracking performance. *Neuropsychologia* 48 (5): 1472–82.

Carlson NR. 2013. *Physiology of Behavior*. Amherst: Pearson.

Carter CS, and van Veen V. 2007. Anterior cingulate cortex and conflict detection: an update of theory and data. *Cogn Affect Behav Neurosci* 7 (4): 367–79.

Catenoix H, Magnin M, Mauguiere F, and Ryvlin P. 2011. Evoked potential study of hippocampal efferent projections in the human brain. *Clin Neurophysiol* 122 (12): 2488–97.

Chantome M, Perruchet P, Hasboun D, Dormont D, Sahel M, Sourour N, Zouaoui A, Marsault C, and Duyme M. 1999. Is there a negative correlation between explicit memory and hippocampal volume? *Neuroimage* 10 (5): 589–95.

Chapman HL, Eramudugolla R, Gavrilescu M, Strudwick MW, Loftus A, Cunnington R, and Mattingley JB. 2010. Neural mechanisms underlying spatial realignment during adaptation to optical wedge prisms. *Neuropsychologia* 48 (9): 2595–2601.

Cheek P, Nikpour L, and Nowlin HD. 2005. Aging well with smart technology. *Nurs Adm Q* 29 (4): 329–38.

Chojnacki AK, Mak GK, and Weiss S. 2009. Identity crisis for adult periventricular neural stem cells: subventricular zone astrocytes, ependymal cells or both? *Nat Rev Neurosci* 10 (2): 153–63.

Cincotti F, Aloise F, Bufalari S, Schalk G, Oriolo G, Cherubini A, Davide F, Babiloni F, Marciani MG, and Mattia D. 2007. Non-invasive brain-computer interface system to operate assistive devices. *Conf Proc IEEE Eng Med Biol Soc*: 2532–35.

Cipriani G, Bianchetti A, and Trabucchi M. 2006. Outcomes of a computer-based cognitive rehabilitation program on Alzheimer's disease patients compared with those on patients affected by mild cognitive impairment. *Arch Gerontol Geriatr* 43 (3): 327–35.

Clark JE, Lanphear AK, and Riddick CC. 1987. The effects of videogame playing on the response selection processing of elderly adults. *J Gerontol* 42 (1): 82–85.

Craik FI, Bialystok E, and Freedman M. 2010. Delaying the onset of Alzheimer disease: bilingualism as a form of cognitive reserve. *Neurology* 75 (19): 1726–29.

Cruts M, van Duijn CM, Backhovens H, Van den Broeck M, Wehnert A, Serneels S, Sherrington R, Hutton M, Hardy J, St. George-Hyslop PH, Hofman A, and Van BC. 1998. Estimation of the genetic contribution of presenilin-1 and -2 mutations in a population-based study of presenile Alzheimer disease. *Hum Mol Genet* 7 (1): 43–51.

Curiati PK, Tamashiro JH, Squarzoni P, Duran FL, Santos LC, Wajngarten M, Leite CC, Vallada H, Menezes PR, Scazufca M, Busatto GF, and Alves TC. 2009. Brain structural variability due to aging and gender in cognitively healthy elders: results from the Sao Paulo Ageing and Health study. *Am J Neuroradiol* 30 (10): 1850–56.

Czaja S, and Lee C. 2007. The impact of aging on access to technology. *Universal Access in the Information Society* 5 (4): 341–49.

Daily Mail. 2010. Patients with locked-in syndrome will soon be able to communicate with mind-reading technology, predicts scientist. September 21.

Dale AM, Liu AK, Fischl BR, Buckner RL, Belliveau JW, Lewine JD, and Halgren E. 2000. Dynamic statistical parametric mapping: combining fMRI and MEG for high-resolution imaging of cortical activity. *Neuron* 26 (1): 55–67.

Danker JF, and Anderson JR. 2010. The ghosts of brain states past: remembering reactivates the brain regions engaged during encoding. *Psychol Bull* 136 (1): 87–102.

Davies HD, Sridhar SB, Newkirk LA, Beaudreau SA, and O'Hara R. 2012. Gender differences in sexual behaviors of AD patients and their relationship to spousal caregiver well-being. *Aging Ment Health* 16 (1): 89–101.

Davies HD, Zeiss AM, Shea EA, and Tinklenberg JR. 1998. Sexuality and intimacy in Alzheimer's patients and their partners. *Sexuality and Disability* 16 (3): 193–203.

Davis SW, Dennis NA, Daselaar SM, Fleck MS, and Cabeza R. 2008. Que PASA? The posterior-anterior shift in aging. *Cereb Cortex* 18 (5): 1201–9.

Dehaene-Lambertz G, Dehaene S, and Hertz-Pannier L. 2002. Functional neuroimaging of speech perception in infants. *Science* 298 (5600): 2013–15.

Dekosky ST, and Scheff SW. 1990. Synapse loss in frontal cortex biopsies in Alzheimer's disease: correlation with cognitive severity. *Ann. Neurol* 27 (5): 457–64.

Deng W, Aimone JB, and Gage FH. 2010. New neurons and new memories: how does adult hippocampal neurogenesis affect learning and memory? *Nat Rev Neurosci* 11 (5): 339–50.

den Heijer T, Geerlings MI, Hoebeek FE, Hofman A, Koudstaal PJ, and Breteler MM. 2006. Use of hippocampal and amygdalar volumes on magnetic resonance imaging to predict dementia in cognitively intact elderly people. *Arch Gen Psychiatry* 63 (1): 57–62.

den Heijer T, Sijens PE, Prins ND, Hofman A, Koudstaal PJ, Oudkerk M, and Breteler MM. 2006. MR spectroscopy of brain white matter in the prediction of dementia. *Neurology* 66 (4): 540–44.

de Vries PM, de Jong BM, Bohning DE, Walker JA, George MS, and Leenders KL. 2009. Changes in cerebral activations during movement execution and imagery after parietal cortex TMS interleaved with 3T MRI. *Brain Res* 1285:58–68.

Dorjgochoo T, Deming SL, Gao YT, Lu W, Zheng Y, Ruan Z, Zheng W, and Shu XO. 2008. History of benign breast disease and risk of breast cancer among women in China: a case-control study. *Cancer Causes Control* 19 (8): 819–28.

Duhamel JR, Colby CL, and Goldberg ME. 1992. The updating of the representation of visual space in parietal cortex by intended eye movements. *Science* 255 (5040): 90–92.

Duthie SJ, Whalley LJ, Collins AR, Leaper S, Berger K, and Deary IJ. 2002. Homocysteine, B vitamin status, and cognitive function in the elderly. *Am J Clin Nutr* 75 (5): 908–13.

Emotiv. 2012. www.emotiv.com.

Encinas JM, Michurina TV, Peunova N, Park JH, Tordo J, Peterson DA, Fishell G, Koulakov A, and Enikolopov G. 2011. Division-coupled astrocytic differentiation and age-related depletion of neural stem cells in the adult hippocampus. *Cell Stem Cell* 8 (5): 566–79.

Erickson KI, Voss MW, Prakash RS, Basak C, Szabo A, Chaddock L, Kim JS, Heo S, Alves H, White SM, Wojcicki TR, Mailey E, Vieira VJ, Martin SA, Pence BD, Woods JA, McAuley E, and Kramer AF. 2011. Exercise training increases size of hippocampus and improves memory. *Proc Natl Acad Sci USA* 108 (7): 3017–22.

Evans DA, Hebert LE, Beckett LA, Scherr PA, Albert MS, Chown MJ, Pilgrim DM, and Taylor JO. 1997. Education and other measures of socioeconomic status and risk of incident Alzheimer disease in a defined population of older persons. *Arch Neurol* 54 (11): 1399–1405.

Eyler LT, Sherzai A, Kaup AR, and Jeste DV. 2011. A review of functional brain imaging correlates of successful cognitive aging. *Biol Psychiatry* 70 (2): 115–22.

Faber-Langendoen K, Morris JC, Knesevich JW, LaBarge E, Miller JP, and Berg L. 1988. Aphasia in senile dementia of the Alzheimer type. *Ann Neurol* 23 (4): 365–70.

Fan J, Stukas S, Wong C, Chan J, May S, DeValle N, Hirsch-Reinshagen V, Wilkinson A, Oda MN, and Wellington CL. 2011. An ABCA1-independent pathway for recycling a poorly lipidated 8.1 nm apolipoprotein E particle from glia. *J Lipid Res* 52 (9): 1605–16.

Fan M, Liu B, Zhou Y, Zhen X, Xu C, and Jiang T. 2010. Cortical thickness is associated with different apolipoprotein E genotypes in healthy elderly adults. *Neurosci Lett* 479 (3): 332–36.

Farina E, Mantovani F, Fioravanti R, Pignatti R, Chiavari L, Imbornone E, Olivotto F, Alberoni M, Mariani C, and Nemni R. 2006. Evaluating two group programmes of cognitive training in mild-to-moderate AD: is there any difference between a "global" stimulation and a "cognitive-specific" one? *Aging Ment Health* 10 (3): 211–18.

Feldman M. 2011. The next step in human brain simulation. *HPC Wire*. July 11.

Fillenbaum GG, Kuchibhatla MN, Hanlon JT, Artz MB, Pieper CF, Schmader KE, Dysken MW, and Gray SL. 2005. Dementia and Alzheimer's disease in community-dwelling elders taking vitamin C and/or vitamin E. *Ann Pharmacother* 39 (12): 2009–14.

Foster HD. 2002. Why the preeminent risk factor in sporadic Alzheimer's disease cannot be genetic. *Med Hypotheses* 59 (1): 57–61.

Fotherby MD, Williams JC, Forster LA, Craner P, and Ferns GA. 2000. Effect of vitamin C on ambulatory blood pressure and plasma lipids in older persons. *J Hypertens* 18 (4): 411–15.

Fratiglioni L, Mangialasche F, and Qiu C. 2010. Brain aging: lessons from community studies. *Nutr Rev* 68 (suppl 2): S119–27.

Friedman R, and Tappen RM. 1991. The effect of planned walking on communication in Alzheimer's disease. *J Am Geriatr Soc* 39 (7): 650–54.

Frisoni GB, Pievani M, Testa C, Sabattoli F, Bresciani L, Bonetti M, Beltramello A, Hayashi KM, Toga AW, and Thompson PM. 2007. The topography of grey matter involvement in early and late onset Alzheimer's disease. *Brain* 130 (3): 720–30.

Fritsch T, Smyth KA, Debanne SM, Petot GJ, and Friedland RP. 2005. Participation in novelty-seeking leisure activities and Alzheimer's disease. *J Geriatr Psychiatry Neurol* 18 (3): 134–41.

Fritsch T, Smyth KA, McClendon MJ, Ogrocki PK, Santillan C, Larsen JD, and Strauss ME. 2005. Associations between dementia/mild cognitive impairment and cognitive performance and activity levels in youth. *J Am Geriatr Soc* 53 (7): 1191–96.

Gabryelewicz T, Styczynska M, Luczywek E, Barczak A, Pfeffer A, Androsiuk W, Choda-kowska-Zebrowska M, Wasiak B, Peplonska B, and Barcikowska M. 2007. The rate of conversion of mild cognitive impairment to dementia: predictive role of depression. *Int J Geriatr Psychiatry* 22 (6): 563–67.

Garrett B. 2011. *Brain & Behavior*. Thousand Oaks, CA: Sage.

Garry PJ, VanderJagt DJ, and Hunt WC. 1987. Ascorbic acid intakes and plasma levels in healthy elderly. *Ann NY Acad Sci* 498: 90–99.

Gautam P, Cherbuin N, Sachdev PS, Wen W, and Anstey KJ. 2011. Relationships between cognitive function and frontal grey matter volumes and thickness in middle aged and early old-aged adults: the PATH Through Life Study. *Neuroimage* 55 (3): 845–55.

Gazzaniga MS. 2012. *Psychological Science* New York: W. W. Norton.

Geldmacher DS, and Whitehouse PJ. 1997. Differential diagnosis of Alzheimer's disease. *Neurology* 48 (5; suppl 6): S2–S9.

Giedd JN. 2004. Structural magnetic resonance imaging of the adolescent brain. *Ann NY Acad Sci* 1021:77–85.

Giovagnoli AR, Erbetta A, Reati F, and Bugiani O. 2008. Differential neuropsychological patterns of frontal variant frontotemporal dementia and Alzheimer's disease in a study of diagnostic concordance. *Neuropsychologia* 46 (5): 1495–1504.

Goedert M, and Spillantini MG. 2006. A century of Alzheimer's disease. *Science* 314 (5800): 777–81.

Gold JJ, Smith CN, Bayley PJ, Shrager Y, Brewer JB, Stark CE, Hopkins RO, and Squire LR. 2006. Item memory, source memory, and the medial temporal lobe: concordant findings from fMRI and memory-impaired patients. *Proc Natl Acad Sci USA* 103 (24): 9351–56.

Goldstein J, Cajko L, Oosterbroek M, Michielsen M, van Houten O, and Salverda F. 1997. Video games and the elderly. *Social Behavior and Personality* 25 (4): 345–52.

Good CD, Johnsrude IS, Ashburner J, Henson RN, Friston KJ, and Frackowiak RS. 2001. A voxel-based morphometric study of ageing in 465 normal adult human brains. *Neuroimage* 14 (1): 21–36.

Gorelick PB, Scuteri A, Black SE, Decarli C, Greenberg SM, Iadecola C, Launer LJ, Laurent S, Lopez OL, Nyenhuis D, Petersen RC, Schneider JA, Tzourio C, Arnett DK, Bennett DA, Chui HC, Higashida RT, Lindquist R, Nilsson PM, Roman GC, Sellke FW, and Seshadri S. 2011. Vascular contributions to cognitive impairment and dementia: a statement for health-care professionals from the American Heart Association/American Stroke Association. *Stroke* 42 (9): 2672–2713.

Grea H, Pisella L, Rossetti Y, Desmurget M, Tilikete C, Grafton S, Prablanc C, and Vighetto A. 2002. A lesion of the posterior parietal cortex disrupts on-line adjustments during aiming movements. *Neuropsychologia* 40 (13): 2471–480.

Greenwood PM, and Parasuraman R. 2010. Neuronal and cognitive plasticity: a neurocognitive framework for ameliorating cognitive aging. *Front Aging Neurosci.* 2:150.

Gregory C, Lough S, Stone V, Erzinclioglu S, Martin L, Baron-Cohen S, and Hodges JR. 2002. Theory of mind in patients with frontal variant frontotemporal dementia and Alzheimer's disease: theoretical and practical implications. *Brain* 125 (4): 752–64.

Grindrod CM, Bilenko NY, Myers EB, and Blumstein SE. 2008. The role of the left inferior frontal gyrus in implicit semantic competition and selection: an event-related fMRI study. *Brain Res* 1229: 167–78.

Guardia-Laguarta C, Pera M, and Lleo A. 2010. Gamma-secretase as a therapeutic target in Alzheimer's disease. *Curr Drug Targets* 11 (4): 506–17.

Gunning-Dixon FM, and Raz N. 2000. The cognitive correlates of white matter abnormalities in normal aging: a quantitative review. *Neuropsychology* 14 (2): 224–32.

Gunther ML, Jackson JC, and Ely EW. 2007. Loss of IQ in the ICU brain injury without the insult. *Med Hypotheses* 69 (6): 1179–82.

Haan MN, and Wallace R. 2004. Can dementia be prevented? Brain aging in a population-based context. *Annu Rev Public Health* 25: 1–24.

Hachinski VC, Lassen NA, and Marshall J. 1974. Multi-infarct dementia: a cause of mental deterioration in the elderly. *Lancet* 2 (7874): 207–10.

Hagberg B, Bauer AB, Poon LW, and Homma A. 2001. Cognitive functioning in centenarians: a coordinated analysis of results from three countries. *J Gerontol B Psychol Sci Soc Sci* 56 (3): 141–51.

Hamilton AC, Martin RC, and Burton PC. 2010. Converging functional magnetic resonance imaging evidence for a role of the left inferior frontal lobe in semantic retention during language comprehension. *Cogn Neuropsychol*: 1–20.

Hansson O, Zetterberg H, Buchhave P, Londos E, Blennow K, and Minthon L. 2006. Association between CSF biomarkers and incipient Alzheimer's disease in patients with mild cognitive impairment: a follow-up study. *Lancet Neurol* 5 (3): 228–34.

Harris SM, Adams MS, Zubatsky M, and White M. 2011. A caregiver perspective of how Alzheimer's disease and related disorders affect couple intimacy. *Aging Ment Health* 15 (8): 950–60.

Harrison FE, and May JM. 2009. Vitamin C function in the brain: vital role of the ascorbate transporter SVCT2. *Free Radic Biol Med* 46 (6): 719–30.

Harrison TM, Weintraub S, Mesulam MM, and Rogalski E. 2012. Superior memory and higher cortical volumes in unusually successful cognitive aging. *Journal of the International Neuropsychological Society* 18: 1–5.

Hassabis D, Chu C, Rees G, Weiskopf N, Molyneux PD, and Maguire EA. 2009. Decoding neuronal ensembles in the human hippocampus. *Curr Biol* 19 (7): 546–54.

Hatanpaa K, Isaacs KR, Shirao T, Brady DR, and Rapoport SI. 1999. Loss of proteins regulating synaptic plasticity in normal aging of the human brain and in Alzheimer disease. *J Neuropathol Exp Neurol* 58 (6): 637–43.

Hayashi K, Ishikawa R, Ye LH, He XL, Takata K, Kohama K, and Shirao T. 1996. Modulatory role of drebrin on the cytoskeleton within dendritic spines in the rat cerebral cortex. *J Neurosci* 16 (22): 7161–70.

Herculano-Houzel S. 2009. The human brain in numbers: a linearly scaled-up primate brain. *Front Hum Neurosci* 3:31.

Hirsch-Reinshagen V, Zhou S, Burgess BL, Bernier L, McIsaac SA, Chan JY, Tansley GH, Cohn JS, Hayden MR, and Wellington CL. 2004. Deficiency of ABCA1 impairs apolipoprotein E metabolism in brain. *J Biol Chem* 279 (39): 41197–41207.

Hochberg LR, Serruya MD, Friehs GM, Mukand JA, Saleh M, Caplan AH, Branner A, Chen D, Penn RD, and Donoghue JP. 2006. Neuronal ensemble control of prosthetic devices by a human with tetraplegia. *Nature* 442 (7099): 164–71.

Hockey R, Gaillard AWK, Coles MGH, North Atlantic Treaty Organization, and Scientific Affairs Division. 1986. *Energetics and Human Information Processing*. Dordrecht: Nijhoff.

Hoffmann T, Bennett S, Koh CL, and McKenna K. 2010. A systematic review of cognitive interventions to improve functional ability in people who have cognitive impairment following stroke. *Top Stroke Rehabil* 17 (2): 99–107.

Holroyd S, Shepherd ML, and Downs JH, III. 2000. Occipital atrophy is associated with visual hallucinations in Alzheimer's disease. *J Neuropsychiatry Clin Neurosci* 12 (1): 25–28.

Howard G, Wagenknecht LE, Cai J, Cooper L, Kraut MA, and Toole JF. 1998. Cigarette smoking and other risk factors for silent cerebral infarction in the general population. *Stroke* 29 (5): 913–17.

Huber K, and Superti-Furga G. 2011. After the grape rush: Sirtuins as epigenetic drug targets in neurodegenerative disorders. *Bioorg Med Chem* 9 (12): 3616–24.

Husain M, and Mehta MA. 2011. Cognitive enhancement by drugs in health and disease. *Trends Cogn Sci* 15 (1): 28–36.

Ikonomovic MD, Klunk WE, Abrahamson EE, Mathis CA, Price JC, Tsopelas ND, Lopresti BJ, Ziolko S, Bi W, Paljug WR, Debnath ML, Hope CE, Isanski BA, Hamilton RL, and Dekosky ST. 2008. Post-mortem correlates of in vivo PiB-PET amyloid imaging in a typical case of Alzheimer's disease. *Brain* 131 (6): 1630–45.

Ingram DK, Cutler RG, Weindruch R, Renquist DM, Knapka JJ, April M, Belcher CT, Clark MA, Hatcherson CD, and Marriott BM. 1990. Dietary restriction and aging: the initiation of a primate study. *J Gerontol.* 45 (5): B148–63.

Institute of Medicine, Food and Nutrition Board. 200l. *Dietary Reference Intakes for Vitamin A, Vitamin K, Arsenic, Boron, Chromium, Copper, Iodine, Iron, Manganese, Molybdenum, Nickel, Silicon, Vanadium and Zinic.* Washington, DC: National Academy Press.

Iqbal K, Alonso AC, Gong CX, Khatoon S, Pei JJ, Wang JZ, and Grundke-Iqbal I. 1998. Mechanisms of neurofibrillary degeneration and the formation of neurofibrillary tangles. *J Neural Transm Suppl* 53:169–80.

Jack CR, Albert MS, Knopman DS, McKhann GM, Sperling RA, Carrillo MC, Thies B, and Phelps CH. 2011. Introduction to the recommendations from the National Institute on Aging–Alzheimer's Association workgroups on diagnostic guidelines for Alzheimer's disease. *Alzheimers Dement* 7 (3): 257–62.

Jacquin A, Aboa-Eboule C, Rouaud O, Osseby GV, Binquet C, Durier J, Moreau T, Bonithon-Kopp C, Giroud M, and Bejot Y. 2011. Prior transient ischemic attack and dementia after subsequent ischemic stroke. *Alzheimer Dis Assoc Disord* 26 (4): 307–13.

Jenkin M, and Harris L. 2009. *Cortical Mechanisms of Vision.* Cambridge: Cambridge University Press.

Jenkins LJ, and Ranganath C. 2010. Prefrontal and medial temporal lobe activity at encoding predicts temporal context memory. *J Neurosci* 30 (46): 15558–65.

Jernigan TL, Archibald SL, Fennema-Notestine C, Gamst AC, Stout JC, Bonner J, and Hesselink JR. 2001. Effects of age on tissues and regions of the cerebrum and cerebellum. *Neurobiol Aging* 22 (4): 581–94.

Jeune B, and Andersen-Ranberg K. 1999. [What can be learned from centenarians?] *Ugeskr Laeger* 161 (46): 6321–25.

Kendziorra K, Wolf H, Meyer PM, Barthel H, Hesse S, Becker GA, Luthardt J, Schildan A, Patt M, Sorger D, Seese A, Gertz HJ, and Sabri O. 2011. Decreased cerebral alpha4beta2* nicotinic acetylcholine receptor availability in patients with mild cognitive impairment and Alzheimer's disease assessed with positron emission tomography. *Eur J Nucl Med Mol Imaging* 38 (3): 515–25.

Kennedy AM, Boyle EM, Traynor O, Walsh T, and Hill AD. 2011. Video gaming enhances psychomotor skills but not visuospatial and perceptual abilities in surgical trainees. *J Surg Educ* 68 (5): 414–20.

Kester MI, van der Vlies AE, Blankenstein MA, Pijnenburg YA, van Elk EJ, Scheltens P, and van der Flier WM. 2009. CSF biomarkers predict rate of cognitive decline in Alzheimer disease. *Neurology* 73 (17): 1353–58.

Kindratenko V. 2011. Trends in high-performance computing. *Comp Sci Eng* 13 (3): 92–95.

Kliegel M, Moor C, and Rott C. 2004. Cognitive status and development in the oldest old: a longitudinal analysis from the Heidelberg Centenarian Study. *Arch Gerontol Geriatr* 39 (2): 143–56.

Knapp M, Thorgrimsen L, Patel A, Spector A, Hallam A, Woods B, and Orrell M. 2006. Cognitive stimulation therapy for people with dementia: cost-effectiveness analysis. *Br J Psychiatry* 188:574–80.

Kolb B, and Wishaw IQ. 2009. *Fundamentals of Human Neuropsychology.* New York: Worth.

Kolb B, Morshead C, Gonzalez C, Kim M, Gregg C, Shingo T, and Weiss S. 2007. Growth factor-stimulated generation of new cortical tissue and functional recovery after stroke damage to the motor cortex of rats. *J Cereb Blood Flow Metab* 27 (5): 983–97.

Komarova NL, and Thalhauser CJ. 2011. High degree of heterogeneity in Alzheimer's disease progression patterns. *PLoS Comput Biol* 7 (11): e1002251.

Krawczyk DC, Michelle MM, and Donovan CM. 2011. A hierarchy for relational reasoning in the prefrontal cortex. *Cortex* 47 (5): 588–97.

Kurzweil R. 2005. Human life: the next generation. *New Scientist.* September 24.

Kwok V, Niu Z, Kay P, Zhou K, Mo L, Jin Z, So KF, and Tan LH. 2011. Learning new color names produces rapid increase in gray matter in the intact adult human cortex. *Proc Natl Acad Sci USA* 108 (16): 6686–88.

Lambourne K, and Tomporowski P. 2010. The effect of exercise-induced arousal on cognitive task performance: a meta-regression analysis. *Brain Res* 1341:12–24.

Landmark K. 2006. [Could intake of vitamins C and E inhibit development of Alzheimer dementia?] *Tidsskr Nor Laegeforen* 126 (2): 159–61.

Lane MA, Ingram DK, Ball SS, and Roth GS. 1997. Dehydroepiandrosterone sulfate: a biomarker of primate aging slowed by calorie restriction. *J Clin Endocrinol Metab* 82 (7): 2093–96.

Lanni C, Lenzken SC, Pascale A, Del Vecchio, I, Racchi M, Pistoia F, and Govoni S. 2008. Cognition enhancers between treating and doping the mind. *Pharmacol Res* 57 (3): 196–213.

Laplagne DA, Esposito MS, Piatti VC, Morgenstern NA, Zhao C, van Praag H, Gage FH, and Schinder AF. 2006. Functional convergence of neurons generated in the developing and adult hippocampus. *PLoS Biol* 4 (12): e409.

Larson EB, Wang L, Bowen JD, McCormick WC, Teri L, Crane P, and Kukull W. 2006. Exercise is associated with reduced risk for incident dementia among persons 65 years of age and older. *Ann Intern Med* 144 (2): 73–81.

Levy-Lahad E, Wijsman EM, Nemens E, Anderson L, Goddard KA, Weber JL, Bird TD, and Schellenberg GD. 1995. A familial Alzheimer's disease locus on chromosome 1. *Science* 269 (5226): 970–73.

Lezak MD. 1995. *Neuropsychological Assessment.* New York: Oxford University Press.

Lin SH, Yu CY, and Pai MC. 2006. The occipital white matter lesions in Alzheimer's disease patients with visual hallucinations. *Clin Imaging* 30 (6): 388–93.

Lind J. 1753. *A Treatise of the Scurvy.* Edinburgh: A. Millar.

Loewenstein DA, Acevedo A, Czaja SJ, and Duara R. 2004. Cognitive rehabilitation of mildly impaired Alzheimer disease patients on cholinesterase inhibitors. *Am J Geriatr Psychiatry* 12 (4): 395–402.

Long J, Li Y, Wang H, Yu T, Pan J, and Li F. 2012. A hybrid brain computer interface to control the direction and speed of a simulated or real wheelchair. *IEEE Trans Neural Syst Rehabil Eng* 20 (5): 720–29.

Lowdon P, Murray A, and Langley P. 2011. Heart rate and blood pressure interactions during attempts to consciously raise or lower heart rate and blood pressure in normotensive subjects. *Physiol Meas* 32 (3): 359–67.

Lynch G, Palmer LC, and Gall CM. 2011. The likelihood of cognitive enhancement. *Pharmacol Biochem Behav* 99 (2): 116–29.

Lynch J, Aughwane P, and Hammond TM. 2010. Video games and surgical ability: a literature review. *J Surg Educ* 67 (3): 184–89.

Macdonald SW, Decarlo CA, and Dixon RA. 2011. Linking biological and cognitive aging: toward improving characterizations of developmental time. *J Gerontol B Psychol Sci Soc Sci* 66 (suppl 1): I59–70.

Madureira S, Canhao P, Guerreiro M, and Ferro JM. 2000. Cognitive and emotional consequences of perimesencephalic subarachnoid hemorrhage. *J Neuro.* 247 (11): 862–67.

Maguire EA, Gadian DG, Johnsrude IS, Good CD, Ashburner J, Frackowiak RS, and Frith CD. 2000. Navigation-related structural change in the hippocampi of taxi drivers. *Proc Natl Acad Sci USA* 97 (8): 4398–4403.

Mahoney DM, Mutschler PH, Tarlow B, and Liss E. 2008. Real world implementation lessons and outcomes from the Worker Interactive Networking (WIN) project: workplace-based online caregiver support and remote monitoring of elders at home. *Telemed J E Health* 14 (3): 224–34.

Maioli F, Coveri M, Pagni P, Chiandetti C, Marchetti C, Ciarrocchi R, Ruggero C, Nativio V, Onesti A, D'Anastasio C, and Pedone V. 2007. Conversion of mild cognitive impairment to dementia in elderly subjects: a preliminary study in a memory and cognitive disorder unit. *Arch Gerontol Geriatr* 44 (suppl 1): 233–41.

Marioni RE, van den Hout A, Valenzuela MJ, Brayne C, and Matthews FE. 2012. Active cognitive lifestyle associates with cognitive recovery and a reduced risk of cognitive decline. *J Alzheimers Dis* 28 (1): 223–30.

Markram H. 2006. The blue brain project. *Nat Rev Neurosci* 7 (2): 153–60.

Marlatt MW, and Lucassen PJ. 2010. Neurogenesis and Alzheimer's disease: biology and pathophysiology in mice and men. *Curr Alzheimer Res* 7 (2): 113–25.

Masterjohn C. 2007. Vitamin D toxicity redefined: vitamin K and the molecular mechanism. *Med Hypotheses* 68 (5): 1026–34.

Mattson MP. 2000. Neuroprotective signaling and the aging brain: take away my food and let me run. *Brain Res* 886 (1–2): 47–53.

Mayeux R. 2003. Epidemiology of neurodegeneration. *Annu Rev Neurosci* 26: 81–104.

Mayeux R, and Stern Y. 2012. Epidemiology of Alzheimer disease. *Cold Spring Harb Perspect Med* 2 (8).

McCarthy RA, Evans JJ, and Hodges JR. 1996. Topographic amnesia: spatial memory disorder, perceptual dysfunction, or category specific semantic memory impairment? *J Neurol Neurosurg Psychiatry* 60 (3): 318–25.

McKhann G, Drachman D, Folstein M, Katzman R, Price D, and Stadlan EM. 1984. Clinical diagnosis of Alzheimer's disease: report of the NINCDS-ADRDA Work Group under the auspices of Department of Health and Human Services Task Force on Alzheimer's Disease. *Neurology* 34 (7): 939–44.

McKhann GM, Knopman DS, Chertkow H, Hyman BT, Jack CR, Kawas CH, Klunk WE, Koroshetz WJ, Manly JJ, Mayeux R, Mohs RC, Morris JC, Rossor MN, Scheltens P, Carrillo MC, Thies B, Weintraub S, and Phelps CH. 2011. The diagnosis of dementia due to Alzheimer's disease: recommendations from the National Institute on Aging–Alzheimer's Association workgroups on diagnostic guidelines for Alzheimer's disease. *Alzheimers Dement* 7 (3): 263–69.

McMorris T, Omporowski P, and Audiffren M. 2009. *Exercise and Cognitive Function.* Chichester, UK: Wiley-Blackwell.

Metitieri T, Zanetti O, Geroldi C, Frisoni GB, De Leo D, Dello BM, Bianchetti A, and Trabucchi M. 2001. Reality orientation therapy to delay outcomes of progression in patients with dementia: a retrospective study. *Clin Rehabil* 15 (5): 471–78.

Miller ER, Pastor-Barriuso R, Dalal D, Riemersma RA, Appel LJ, and Guallar E. 2005. Meta-analysis: high dosage vitamin E supplementation may increase all-cause mortality. *Ann of Intern Med* 142:37–46.

Moreau F, Jeerakathil T, Coutts SB, and FRCPC for the ASPIRE Investigators. 2012. Patients referred for TIA may still have persisting neurological deficits. *Can J Neurol Sci* 39 (2): 170–73.

Mufson EJ, Binder L, Counts SE, Dekosky ST, de Toledo-Morrell L, Ginsberg SD, Ikonomovic MD, Perez SE, and Scheff SW. 2012. Mild cognitive impairment: pathology and mechanisms. *Acta Neuropathol* 123 (1): 13–30.

Muller DP. 2010. Vitamin E and neurological function. *Mol Nutr Food Res* 54 (5): 710–18.

Murray AD, Staff RT, McNeil CJ, Salarirad S, Ahearn TS, Mustafa N, and Whalley LJ. 2011. The balance between cognitive reserve and brain imaging biomarkers of cerebrovascular and Alzheimer's diseases. *Brain.* December 7.

Nadolne MJ, and Stringer AY. 2001. Ecologic validity in neuropsychological assessment: prediction of wayfinding. *J Int Neuropsychol Soc* 7 (6): 675–82.

National Institutes of Health, U.S. Department of Health and Human Services, U.S Department of State, and National Institute of Aging. 2007. *Why Population Aging Matters: A Global Perspective.*

Nelson PT, Alafuzoff I, Bigio EH, Bouras C, Braak H, Cairns NJ, Castellani RJ, Crain BJ, Davies P, Tredici KD, Duyckaerts C, Frosch MP, Haroutunian V, Hof PR, Hulette CM, Hyman BT, Iwatsubo T, Jellinger KA, Jicha GA, Kovari E, Kukull WA, Leverenz JB, Love S, Mackenzie IR, Mann DM, Masliah E, McKee AC, Montine TJ, Morris JC, Schneider JA, Sonnen JA, Thal DR, Trojanowski JQ, Troncoso JC, Wisniewski T, Woltjer RL, and Beach TG. 2012. Correlation of Alzheimer disease neuropathologic changes with cognitive status: a review of the literature. *J Neuropathol Exp Neurol* 71 (5): 362–81.

Nichol KE, Parachikova AI, and Cotman CW. 2007. Three weeks of running wheel exposure improves cognitive performance in the aged Tg2576 mouse. *Behav Brain Res* 184 (2): 124–32.

Ohlendorf S, Sprenger A, Speck O, Glauche V, Haller S, and Kimmig H. 2010. Visual motion, eye motion, and relative motion: a parametric fMRI study of functional specializations of smooth pursuit eye movement network areas. *J Vis* 10 (14): 21.

Olazaran-Rodriguez J, Cruz-Orduna I, and Jimenez-Martin F. 2004. Donepezil therapy in patients with vascular and post-traumatic cognitive impairment: some clinical observations. *Revista de Neurologia* 38 (10): 938–43.

Orrell M, Spector A, Thorgrimsen L, and Woods B. 2005. A pilot study examining the effectiveness of maintenance cognitive stimulation therapy (MCST) for people with dementia. *Int J Geriatr Psychiatry* 20 (5): 446–51.

Owen AM, and Coleman MR. 2008. Using neuroimaging to detect awareness in disorders of consciousness. *Funct Neurol* 23 (4): 189–94.

Pallier C, Dehaene S, Poline JB, LeBihan D, Argenti AM, Dupoux E, and Mehler J. 2003. Brain imaging of language plasticity in adopted adults: can a second language replace the first? *Cereb Cortex* 13 (2): 155–61.

Parent MB, Krebs-Kraft DL, Ryan JP, Wilson JS, Harenski C, and Hamann S. 2011. Glucose administration enhances fMRI brain activation and connectivity related to episodic memory encoding for neutral and emotional stimuli. *Neuropsychologia* 49 (5): 1052–66.

Park DC, and Reuter-Lorenz P. 2009. The adaptive brain: aging and neurocognitive scaffolding. *Annu Rev Psychol* 60:173–96.

Partridge BJ, Bell SK, Lucke JC, Yeates S, and Hall WD. 2011. Smart drugs "as common as coffee": media hype about neuroenhancement. *PLoS One* 6 (11): e28416.

Pedersen PM, Jorgensen HS, Nakayama H, Raaschou HO, and Olsen TS. 1995. Aphasia in acute stroke: incidence, determinants, and recovery. *Ann Neurol* 38 (4): 659–66.

Pendlebury ST. 2009. Stroke-related dementia: rates, risk factors and implications for future research. *Maturitas* 64 (3): 165–71.

Pendlebury ST, and Rothwell PM. 2009. Prevalence, incidence, and factors associated with pre-stroke and post-stroke dementia: a systematic review and meta-analysis. *Lancet Neurol* 8 (11): 1006–18.

Pendlebury ST, and Rothwell PM. 2009. Risk of recurrent stroke, other vascular events and dementia after transient ischaemic attack and stroke. *Cerebrovasc Dis* 27 (suppl 3): 1–11.

Pendlebury ST, Wadling S, Silver LE, Mehta Z, and Rothwell PM. 2011. Transient cognitive impairment in TIA and minor stroke. *Stroke* 42 (11): 3116–21.

Pereira AC, Huddleston DE, Brickman AM, Sosunov AA, Hen R, McKhann GM, Sloan R, Gage FH, Brown TR, and Small SA. 2007. An in vivo correlate of exercise-induced neurogenesis in the adult dentate gyrus. *Proc Natl Acad Sci USA* 104 (13): 5638–43.

Persson J, and Nyberg L. 2006. Altered brain activity in healthy seniors: what does it mean? *Prog Brain Res* 157:45–56.

Petersen RC, Thomas RG, Grundman M, Bennett D, Doody R, Ferris S, Galasko D, Jin S, Kaye J, Levey A, Pfeiffer E, Sano M, van Dyck CH, and Thal LJ. 2005. Vitamin E and donepezil for the treatment of mild cognitive impairment. *N Engl J Med* 352 (23): 2379–88.

Pettersen JA, Sathiyamoorthy G, Gao FQ, Szilagyi G, Nadkarni NK, St George-Hyslop P, Rogaeva E, and Black SE. 2008. Microbleed topography, leukoaraiosis, and cognition in probable Alzheimer disease from the Sunnybrook dementia study. *Arch Neurol* 65 (6): 790–95.

Piefke M, Onur OA, and Fink GR. 2010. Aging-related changes of neural mechanisms underlying visual-spatial working memory. *Neurobiol Aging* 33 (7): 1284–97.

Price JL, McKeel DW, Buckles VD, Roe CM, Xiong C, Grundman M, Hansen LA, Petersen RC, Parisi JE, Dickson DW, Smith CD, Davis DG, Schmitt FA, Markesbery WR, Kaye J, Kurlan R, Hulette C, Kurland BF, Higdon R, Kukull W, and Morris JC. 2009. Neuropathology of nondemented aging: presumptive evidence for preclinical Alzheimer disease. *Neurobiol Aging* 30 (7): 1026–36.

Price JL, and Morris JC. 1999. Tangles and plaques in nondemented aging and "preclinical" Alzheimer's disease. *Ann Neurol* 45 (3): 358–68.

Price TR, Manolio TA, Kronmal RA, Kittner SJ, Yue NC, Robbins J, Anton-Culver H, and O'Leary DH. 1997. Silent brain infarction on magnetic resonance imaging and neurological abnormalities in community-dwelling older adults: the Cardiovascular Health Study, CHS Collaborative Research Group. *Stroke* 28 (6): 1158–64.

Raber J, Huang Y, and Ashford JW. 2004. ApoE genotype accounts for the vast majority of AD risk and AD pathology. *Neurobiol Aging* 25 (5): 641–50.

Ramirez-Amaya V, Marrone DF, Gage FH, Worley PF, and Barnes CA. 2006. Integration of new neurons into functional neural networks. *J Neurosci* 26 (47): 12237–41.

Rando TA. 2006. Stem cells, ageing and the quest for immortality. *Nature* 441 (7097): 1080–86.

Rando TA, and Chang HY. 2012. Aging, rejuvenation, and epigenetic reprogramming: resetting the aging clock. *Cell* 148 (1–2): 46–57.

Raux G, Guyant-Marechal L, Martin C, Bou J, Penet C, Brice A, Hannequin D, Frebourg T, and Campion D. 2005. Molecular diagnosis of autosomal dominant early onset Alzheimer's disease: an update. *J Med Genet* 42 (10): 793–95.

Raz N, Gunning-Dixon FM, Head D, Dupuis JH, and Acker JD. 1998. Neuroanatomical correlates of cognitive aging: evidence from structural magnetic resonance imaging. *Neuropsychology* 12 (1): 95–114.

Raz N, Lindenberger U, Rodrigue KM, Kennedy KM, Head D, Williamson A, Dahle C, Gerstorf D, and Acker JD. 2005. Regional brain changes in aging healthy adults: general trends, individual differences and modifiers. *Cereb Cortex* 15 (11): 1676–89.

Raz N, Williamson A, Gunning-Dixon F, Head D, and Acker JD. 2000. Neuroanatomical and cognitive correlates of adult age differences in acquisition of a perceptual-motor skill. *Microsc Res Tech* 51 (1): 85–93.

Reiman E, Lopera F, Langbaum J, Fleisher A, Ayutyanont N, Quiroz Y, Jakimovich L, Langlois C, and Tariot P. 2012. The Alzheimer's prevention initiative. Paper presented at Alzheimer's Association International Conference.

Reitz C, Bos MJ, Hofman A, Koudstaal PJ, and Breteler MM. 2008. Prestroke cognitive performance, incident stroke, and risk of dementia: the Rotterdam Study. *Stroke* 39 (1): 36–41.

Relkin N, Bettger L, Tsakanikas D, and Ravdin L. 2012. Three year follow-up on the IVIG for Alzheimer's Phase II Study. Paper presented at Alzheimer's Association International Conference.

Resnick SM, Goldszal AF, Davatzikos C, Golski S, Kraut MA, Metter EJ, Bryan RN, and Zonderman AB. 2000. One-year age changes in MRI brain volumes in older adults. *Cereb Cortex* 10 (5): 464–72.

Reuter-Lorenz PA, and Lustig C. 2005. Brain aging: reorganizing discoveries about the aging mind. *Curr Opin Neurobiol* 15 (2): 245–51.

Revill KP, Karnath HO, and Rorden C. 2011. Distinct anatomy for visual search and bisection: a neuroimaging study. *Neuroimage* 57 (2): 476–81.

Richard T, Pawlus AD, Iglesias ML, Pedrot E, Waffo-Teguo P, Merillon JM, and Monti JP. 2011. Neuroprotective properties of resveratrol and derivatives. *Ann NY Acad Sci* 1215:103–8.

Ritchie AE. 2004. *The a1-antichymotrypsin-51bp promoter polymorphism: functional activity and its role in Alzheimer's disease.* PhD thesis. University of Nottingham.

Ritchie K, and Kildea D. 1995. Is senile dementia "age-related" or "ageing-related"? Evidence from meta-analysis of dementia prevalence in the oldest old. *Lancet* 346 (8980): 931–34.

Rodrigue KM, and Raz N. 2004. Shrinkage of the entorhinal cortex over five years predicts memory performance in healthy adults. *J Neurosci* 24 (4): 956–63.

Rogaev EI, Sherrington R, Rogaeva EA, Levesque G, Ikeda M, Liang Y, Chi H, Lin C, Holman K, and Tsuda T. 1995. Familial Alzheimer's disease in kindreds with missense mutations in a gene on chromosome 1 related to the Alzheimer's disease type 3 gene. *Nature* 376 (6543): 775–78.

Rolland Y, Rival L, Pillard F, Lafont C, Rivere D, Albarede J, and Vellas B. 2000. Feasibility of regular physical exercise for patients with moderate to severe Alzheimer disease. *J Nutr Health Aging* 4 (2): 109–13.

Roth GS, Lesnikov V, Lesnikov M, Ingram DK, and Lane MA. 2001. Dietary caloric restriction prevents the age-related decline in plasma melatonin levels of rhesus monkeys. *J Clin Endocrinol Metab* 86 (7): 3292–95.

Saposnik G, Cote R, Rochon PA, Mamdani M, Liu Y, Raptis S, Kapral MK, and Black SE. 2011. Care and outcomes in patients with ischemic stroke with and without preexisting dementia. *Neurology* 77 (18): 1664–73.

Schacter DL, Curran T, Reiman EM, Chen K, Bandy DJ, and Frost JT. 1999. Medial temporal lobe activation during episodic encoding and retrieval: a PET study. *Hippocampus* 9 (5): 575–81.

Scherder EJ, Van PJ, Deijen JB, Van Der KS, Orlebeke JF, Burgers I, Devriese PP, Swaab DF, and Sergeant JA. 2005. Physical activity and executive functions in the elderly with mild cognitive impairment. *Aging Ment Health* 9 (3): 272–80.

Schneider C. 2005. Chemistry and biology of vitamin E. *Mol Nutr Food Res* 49 (1): 7–30.

Schulte JN, and Yarasheski KE. 2001. Effects of resistance training on the rate of muscle protein synthesis in frail elderly people. *Int J Sport Nutr Exerc Metab* 11 (suppl): S111–18.

Schweizer TA, Ware J, Fischer CE, Craik FI, and Bialystok E. 2011. Bilingualism as a contributor to cognitive reserve: Evidence from brain atrophy in Alzheimer's disease. *Cortex* 48 (8): 991–96.

Sherrington R, Rogaev EI, Liang Y, Rogaeva EA, Levesque G, Ikeda M, Chi H, Lin C, Li G, Holman K, Tsuda T, Mar L, Foncin JF, Bruni AC, Montesi MP, Sorbi S, Rainero I, Pinessi L, Nee L, Chumakov I, Pollen D, Brookes A, Sanseau P, Polinsky RJ, Wasco W, Da Silva HA, Haines JL, Perkicak-Vance MA, Tanzi RE, Roses AD, Fraser PE, Rommens JM, and St. George-Hyslop PH. 1995. Cloning of a gene bearing missense mutations in early-onset familial Alzheimer's disease. *Nature* 375 (6534): 754–60.

Silverman DH, Small GW, Chang CY, Lu CS, Kung De Aburto MA, Chen W, Czernin J, Rapoport SI, Pietrini P, Alexander GE, Schapiro MB, Jagust WJ, Hoffman JM, Welsh-Bohmer KA, Alavi A, Clark CM, Salmon E, de Leon MJ, Mielke R, Cummings JL, Kowell AP, Gambhir SS, Hoh CK, and Phelps ME. 2001. Positron emission tomography in evaluation of dementia: regional brain metabolism and long-term outcome. *JAMA* 286 (17): 2120–27.

Simonelli C, Tripodi F, Rossi R, Fabrizi A, Lembo D, Cosmi V, and Pierleoni L. 2008. The influence of caregiver burden on sexual intimacy and marital satisfaction in couples with an Alzheimer spouse. *Int J Clin Pract* 62 (1): 47–52.

Siren AL, Radyushkin K, Boretius S, Kammer D, Riechers CC, Natt O, Sargin D, Watanabe T, Sperling S, Michaelis T, Price J, Meyer B, Frahm J, and Ehrenreich H. 2006. Global brain atrophy after unilateral parietal lesion and its prevention by erythropoietin. *Brain* 129 (2): 480–89.

Sirintrapun SJ, and Cimic A. 2012. Dynamic nonrobotic telemicroscopy via Skype: a cost effective solution to teleconsultation. *J Pathol Inform* 3:28.

Sitzer DI, Twamley EW, and Jeste DV. 2006. Cognitive training in Alzheimer's disease: a meta-analysis of the literature. *Acta Psychiatr Scand* 114 (2): 75–90.

Smyth KA, Fritsch T, Cook TB, McClendon MJ, Santillan CE, and Friedland RP. 2004. Worker functions and traits associated with occupations and the development of AD. *Neurology* 63 (3): 498–503.

Sobel BP. 2001. Bingo vs. physical intervention in stimulating short-term cognition in Alzheimer's disease patients. *Am J Alzheimers Dis Other Demen* 16 (2): 115–20.

Sole-Padulles C, Bartres-Faz D, Junque C, Vendrell P, Rami L, Clemente IC, Bosch B, Villar A, Bargallo N, Jurado MA, Barrios M, and Molinuevo JL. 2009. Brain structure and function related to cognitive reserve variables in normal aging, mild cognitive impairment and Alzheimer's disease. *Neurobiol Aging* 30 (7): 1114–24.

Sperling R, Donohue M, and Aisen P. 2012. The A4 trial: anti-amyloid treatment of asymptomatic Alzheimer's disease. Paper presented at Alzheimer's Association International Conference.

Statistics Canada. 2004. *Canadian Community Health Survey, Nurition.*

Stern Y, Blumen HM, Rich LW, Richards A, Herzberg G, and Gopher D. 2011. Space Fortress game training and executive control in older adults: a pilot intervention. *Neuropsychol Dev Cogn B Aging Neuropsychol Cogn* 18 (6): 653–77.

Stern Y, Gurland B, Tatemichi TK, Tang MX, Wilder D, and Mayeux R. 1994. Influence of education and occupation on the incidence of Alzheimer's disease. *JAMA* 271 (13): 1004–10.

Stern Y, Habeck C, Moeller J, Scarmeas N, Anderson KE, Hilton HJ, Flynn J, Sackeim H, and Van HR. 2005. Brain networks associated with cognitive reserve in healthy young and old adults. *Cereb Cortex* 15 (4): 394–402.

Stranahan AM, Salas-Vega S, Jiam NT, and Gallagher M. 2011. Interference with reelin signaling in the lateral entorhinal cortex impairs spatial memory. *Neurobiol Learn Mem* 96 (2): 150–55.

Stuss DT, and Alexander MP. 2000. Executive functions and the frontal lobes: a conceptual view. *Psychol Res* 63 (3–4): 289–98.

Sultana R, Banks WA, and Butterfield DA. 2010. Decreased levels of PSD95 and two associated proteins and increased levels of BCl2 and caspase 3 in hippocampus from subjects with amnestic mild cognitive impairment: insights into their potential roles for loss of synapses and memory, accumulation of Abeta, and neurodegeneration in a prodromal stage of Alzheimer's disease. *J Neurosci Res* 88 (3): 469–77.

Svoboda E. 2011. *Smart Aging.* Toronto: Baycrest Innovation & Research.

Svoboda E, Richards B, Leach L, and Mertens V. 2012. PDA and smartphone use by individuals with moderate-to-severe memory impairment: application of a theory-driven training programme. *Neuropsychol Rehabil* 22 (3): 408–27.

Tarraga L, Boada M, Modinos G, Espinosa A, Diego S, Morera A, Guitart M, Balcells J, Lopez OL, and Becker JT. 2006. A randomised pilot study to assess the efficacy of an interactive, multimedia tool of cognitive stimulation in Alzheimer's disease. *J Neurol Neurosurg Psychiatry* 77 (10): 1116–21.

Thalhauser CJ, and Komarova NL. 2012. Alzheimer's disease: rapid and slow progression. *J R Soc Interface* 9 (66): 119–26.

Tippett WJ, and Black SE. 2008. Regional cerebral blood flow correlates of visuospatial tasks in Alzheimer's disease. *J Int Neuropsychol Soc* 14 (6): 1034–45.

Tippett WJ, Krajewski A, and Sergio LE. 2007. Visuomotor integration is compromised in Alzheimer's disease patients reaching for remembered targets. *Eur Neurol* 58 (1): 1–11.

Tippett WJ, and Sergio LE. 2006. Visuomotor integration is impaired in early stage Alzheimer's disease. *Brain Res* 1102 (1): 92–102.

Tippett WJ, Sergio LE, and Black SE. 2012. Compromised visually guided motor control in individuals with Alzheimer's disease: Can reliable distinctions be observed? *J Clin Neurosci* 19 (5): 655–60.

Tomlinson BE, Blessed G, and Roth M. 1970. Observations on the brains of demented old people. *J Neurol Sci* 11 (3): 205–42.

Tomporowski PD. 2003. Effects of acute bouts of exercise on cognition. *Acta Psychol (Amst)* 112 (3): 297–324.

Torres A. 2008. Cognitive effects of videogames on older people. *Proc 7th ICDVRAT with ArtAbilitation*: 191–98.

Ueki A, Shinjo H, Shimode H, Nakajima T, and Morita Y. 2001. Factors associated with mortality in patients with early-onset Alzheimer's disease: a five-year longitudinal study. *Int J Geriatr Psychiatry* 16 (8): 810–15.

Usui N, Haji T, Maruyama M, Katsuyama N, Uchida S, Hozawa A, Omori K, Tsuji I, Kawashima R, and Taira M. 2009. Cortical areas related to performance of WAIS Digit Symbol Test: a functional imaging study. *Neurosci Lett* 463 (1): 1–5.

van Gelder BM, Tijhuis MA, Kalmijn S, Giampaoli S, Nissinen A, and Kromhout D. 2004. Physical activity in relation to cognitive decline in elderly men: the FINE Study. *Neurology* 63 (12): 2316–21.

Van Kampen JM, and Robertson HA. 2005. A possible role for dopamine D3 receptor stimulation in the induction of neurogenesis in the adult rat substantia nigra. *Neuroscience* 136 (2): 381–86.

Van PC. 2004. Relationship between hippocampal volume and memory ability in healthy individuals across the lifespan: review and meta-analysis. *Neuropsychologia* 42 (10): 1394–1413.

Van PC, Plante E, Davidson PS, Kuo TY, Bajuscak L, and Glisky EL. 2004. Memory and executive function in older adults: relationships with temporal and prefrontal gray matter volumes and white matter hyperintensities. *Neuropsychologia* 42 (10): 1313–35.

Vaughan TM, McFarland DJ, Schalk G, Sarnacki WA, Krusienski DJ, Sellers EW, and Wolpaw JR. 2006. The Wadsworth BCI Research and Development Program: at home with BCI. *IEEE Trans Neural Syst Rehabil Eng* 14 (2): 229–33.

Verghese J, Lipton RB, Katz MJ, Hall CB, Derby CA, Kuslansky G, Ambrose AF, Sliwinski M, and Buschke H. 2003. Leisure activities and the risk of dementia in the elderly. *N Engl J Med* 348 (25): 2508–16.

Vermeer SE, den Heijer T, Koudstaal PJ, Oudkerk M, Hofman A, and Breteler MM. 2003. Incidence and risk factors of silent brain infarcts in the population-based Rotterdam Scan Study. *Stroke* 34 (2): 392–96.

Vermeer SE, Koudstaal PJ, Oudkerk M, Hofman A, and Breteler MM. 2002. Prevalence and risk factors of silent brain infarcts in the population-based Rotterdam Scan Study. *Stroke* 33 (1): 21–25.

Villacorta L, Graca-Souza AV, Ricciarelli R, Zingg JM, and Azzi A. 2003. Alpha-tocopherol induces expression of connective tissue growth factor and antagonizes tumor necrosis factor-alpha-mediated downregulation in human smooth muscle cells. *Circ Res* 92 (1): 104–10.

Visser M, and Lambon Ralph MA. 2011. Differential contributions of bilateral ventral anterior temporal lobe and left anterior superior temporal gyrus to semantic processes. *J Cogn Neurosci* 23 (10): 3121–31.

Voelbel GT, Genova HM, Chiaravalotti ND, and Hoptman MJ. 2012. Diffusion tensor imaging of traumatic brain injury review: implications for neurorehabilitation. *NeuroRehabilitation* 31 (3): 281–93.

Voelcker-Rehage C. 2008. Motor-skill learning in older adults—a review of studies on age-related differences. *European Review of Aging and Physical Activity* 5 (1): 5–16.

Voineskos AN, Rajji TK, Lobaugh NJ, Miranda D, Shenton ME, Kennedy JL, Pollock BG, and Mulsant BH. 2010. Age-related decline in white matter tract integrity and cognitive performance: a DTI tractography and structural equation modeling study. *Neurobiol Aging* 33 (1): 21–34.

Wade DT, Hewer RL, David RM, and Enderby PM. 1986. Aphasia after stroke: natural history and associated deficits. *J Neurol Neurosurg Psychiatry* 49 (1): 11–16.

Wahrle SE, Jiang H, Parsadanian M, Kim J, Li A, Knoten A, Jain S, Hirsch-Reinshagen V, Wellington CL, Bales KR, Paul SM, and Holtzman DM. 2008. Overexpression of ABCA1 reduces amyloid deposition in the PDAPP mouse model of Alzheimer disease. *J Clin Invest* 118 (2): 671–82.

Wahrle SE, Jiang H, Parsadanian M, Legleiter J, Han X, Fryer JD, Kowalewski T, and Holtzman DM. 2004. ABCA1 is required for normal central nervous system apoE levels and for lipidation of astrocyte-secreted apoE. *J Biol Chem* 279 (39): 40987–93.

Walle T, Hsieh F, DeLegge MH, Oatis JE, and Walle UK. 2004. High absorption but very low bioavailability of oral resveratrol in humans. *Drug Metab Dispos* 32 (12): 1377–82.

Ward NS, and Frackowiak RS. 2003. Age-related changes in the neural correlates of motor performance. *Brain* 126 (4): 873–88.

Weiss B. 2007. Can endocrine disruptors influence neuroplasticity in the aging brain? *Neurotoxicology* 28 (5): 938–50.

Williams K, Arthur A, Niedens M, Moushey L, and Hutfles L. 2012. In-home monitoring support for dementia caregivers: a feasibility study. *Clin Nurs Res.* September 20.

Williamson C, Alcantar O, Rothlind J, Cahn-Weiner D, Miller BL, and Rosen HJ. 2010. Standardised measurement of self-awareness deficits in FTD and AD. *J Neurol Neurosurg Psychiatry* 81 (2): 140–45.

Wilson RS, Beckett LA, Barnes LL, Schneider JA, Bach J, Evans DA, and Bennett DA. 2002. Individual differences in rates of change in cognitive abilities of older persons. *Psychol Aging* 17 (2): 179–93.

Wingfield A, and Grossman M. 2006. Language and the aging brain: patterns of neural compensation revealed by functional brain imaging. *J Neurophysiol* 96 (6): 2830–39.

Wolpaw JR. 2007. Brain-computer interfaces as new brain output pathways. *J Physiol* 579 (3): 613–19.

Xu J, Kobayashi S, Yamaguchi S, Iijima K, Okada K, and Yamashita K. 2000. Gender effects on age-related changes in brain structure. *Am J Neuroradiol* 21 (1): 112–18.

Yoshikawa G, Momiyama T, Oya S, Takai K, Tanaka J, Higashiyama S, Saito N, Kirino T, and Kawahara N. 2010. Induction of striatal neurogenesis and generation of region-specific functional mature neurons after ischemia by growth factors. Laboratory investigation. *J Neurosurg* 113 (4): 835–50.

Zanetti O, Frisoni GB, De LD, Dello BM, Bianchetti A, and Trabucchi M. 1995. Reality orientation therapy in Alzheimer disease: useful or not? A controlled study. *Alzheimer Dis Assoc Disord* 9 (3): 132–38.

Zeba AN, Sorgho H, Rouamba N, Zongo I, Rouamba J, Guiguemde RT, Hamer DH, Mokhtar N, and Ouedraogo JB. 2008. Major reduction of malaria morbidity with combined vitamin A and zinc supplementation in young children in Burkina Faso: a randomized double blind trial. *Nutr J* 7:7.

Zeiss AM, Davies HD, Wood M, and Tinklenberg JR. 1990. The incidence and correlates of erectile problems in patients with Alzheimer's disease. *Arch Sex Behav* 19 (4): 325–31.

Zhou B, Nakatani E, Teramukai S, Nagai Y, and Fukushima M. 2012. Risk classification in mild cognitive impairment patients for developing Alzheimer's disease. *J Alzheimers Dis* 30 (2): 367–75.

Zhou X, and Merzenich MM. 2009. Developmentally degraded cortical temporal processing restored by training. *Nat Neurosci* 12 (1): 26–28.

Zierhut K, Bogerts B, Schott B, Fenker D, Walter M, Albrecht D, Steiner J, Schutze H, Northoff G, Duzel E, and Schiltz K. 2010. The role of hippocampus dysfunction in deficient memory encoding and positive symptoms in schizophrenia. *Psychiatry Res* 183 (3): 187–94.

Zittermann A, Schleithoff SS, and Koerfer R. 2005. Putting cardiovascular disease and vitamin D insufficiency into perspective. *Br J Nutr* 94 (4): 483–92.

Zitterman A, Schleithoff SS, and Koerfer R. 2006. Markers of bone metabolism in congestive heart failure. *Clin Chim Acta* 366 (1–2): 27–36.

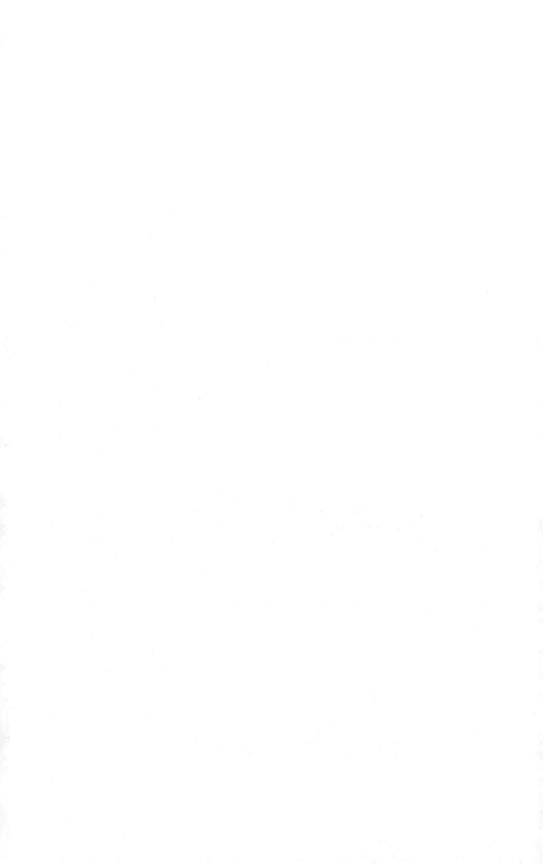

INDEX

ABOUT THE AUTHOR

William J. Tippett, PhD, is assistant professor at the University of Northern British Columbia where he is the principal investigator, founder, and director of the Brain Research Unit and is also an associate member of the Centre for Stroke Recovery with his affiliation held at Sunnybrook Health Sciences Centre, Toronto, Ontario. He is an active researcher and is currently examining how cognitive stimulation programs can alter and change the course of an illness for individuals experiencing dementia-related disturbances and stroke-related injury. He is an active speaker, who has presented at the Society for Neuroscience conference, the British Columbia's Annual Psychogeriatric Conference, and at the Alzheimer's Association International Conference.